Personalized Medicine in Orthopaedics

Personalized Medicine in Orthopaedics

Editors

Arne Kienzle
Henrik Bäcker

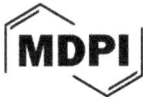

Basel • Beijing • Wuhan • Barcelona • Belgrade • Novi Sad • Cluj • Manchester

Editors
Arne Kienzle
Charité University Hospital Berlin
Berlin
Germany

Henrik Bäcker
Auckland City Hospital
Auckland
New Zealand

Editorial Office
MDPI
St. Alban-Anlage 66
4052 Basel, Switzerland

This is a reprint of articles from the Special Issue published online in the open access journal *Journal of Personalized Medicine* (ISSN 2075-4426) (available at: https://www.mdpi.com/journal/jpm/special_issues/personalized_medicine_orthopaedic).

For citation purposes, cite each article independently as indicated on the article page online and as indicated below:

Lastname, A.A.; Lastname, B.B. Article Title. *Journal Name* **Year**, *Volume Number*, Page Range.

ISBN 978-3-7258-1215-8 (Hbk)
ISBN 978-3-7258-1216-5 (PDF)
doi.org/10.3390/books978-3-7258-1216-5

© 2024 by the authors. Articles in this book are Open Access and distributed under the Creative Commons Attribution (CC BY) license. The book as a whole is distributed by MDPI under the terms and conditions of the Creative Commons Attribution-NonCommercial-NoDerivs (CC BY-NC-ND) license.

Contents

Kunhyung Bae, Gisu Kim, Amaal M. Aldosari, Yeonji Gim and Yoon Hae Kwak
Sterile Silicone Ring Tourniquets in Limb Surgery: A Prospective Clinical Trial in Pediatric Patients Undergoing Orthopedic Surgery
Reprinted from: *J. Pers. Med.* **2023**, *13*, 979, doi:10.3390/jpm13060979 1

So June Hwang, Chiwon Ahn and Moonho Won
Comparing the 30-Day Mortality for Hip Fractures in Patients with and without COVID-19: An Updated Meta-Analysis
Reprinted from: *J. Pers. Med.* **2023**, *13*, 669, doi:10.3390/jpm13040669 12

Carlo Biz, Mariachiara Cerchiaro, Elisa Belluzzi, Elena Bortolato, Alessandro Rossin, Antonio Berizzi and Pietro Ruggieri
Treatment of Distal Radius Fractures with Bridging External Fixator with Optional Percutaneous K-Wires: What Are the Right Indications for Patient Age, Gender, Dominant Limb and Injury Pattern?
Reprinted from: *J. Pers. Med.* **2022**, *12*, 1532, doi:10.3390/jpm12091532 26

Carsten Y. W. Heimer, Chia H. Wu, Carsten Perka, Sebastian Hardt, Friedemann Göhler, Tobias Winkler and Henrik C. Bäcker
The Impact of Hip Dysplasia on CAM Impingement
Reprinted from: *J. Pers. Med.* **2022**, *12*, 1129, doi:10.3390/jpm12071129 42

Henrik C. Bäcker, Kathi Thiele, Chia H. Wu, Philipp Moroder, Ulrich Stöckle and Karl F. Braun
Distal Radius Fracture with Ipsilateral Elbow Dislocation: A Rare but Challenging Injury
Reprinted from: *J. Pers. Med.* **2022**, *12*, 1097, doi:10.3390/jpm12071097 50

Carsten Y. W. Heimer, Chia H. Wu, Carsten Perka, Sebastian Hardt, Friedemann Göhler and Henrik C. Bäcker
The Impact of the Laterality on Radiographic Outcomes of the Bernese Periacetabular Osteotomy
Reprinted from: *J. Pers. Med.* **2022**, *12*, 1072, doi:10.3390/jpm12071072 57

Simon Kwoon-Ho Chow, Marloes van Mourik, Vivian Wing-Yin Hung, Ning Zhang, Michelle Meng-Chen Li, Ronald Man-Yeung Wong, et al.
HR-pQCT for the Evaluation of Muscle Quality and Intramuscular Fat Infiltration in Ageing Skeletal Muscle
Reprinted from: *J. Pers. Med.* **2022**, *12*, 1016, doi:10.3390/jpm12061016 69

Yi Ren, Lara Biedermann, Clemens Gwinner, Carsten Perka and Arne Kienzle
Serum and Synovial Markers in Patients with Rheumatoid Arthritis and Periprosthetic Joint Infection
Reprinted from: *J. Pers. Med.* **2022**, *12*, 810, doi:10.3390/jpm12050810 81

Bo-kyeong Kang, Yelin Han, Jaehoon Oh, Jongwoo Lim, Jongbin Ryu, Myeong Seong Yoon, et al.
Automatic Segmentation for Favourable Delineation of Ten Wrist Bones on Wrist Radiographs Using Convolutional Neural Network
Reprinted from: *J. Pers. Med.* **2022**, *12*, 776, doi:10.3390/jpm12050776 91

Carlo Biz, Davide Scucchiari, Assunta Pozzuoli, Elisa Belluzzi, Nicola Luigi Bragazzi,
Antonio Berizzi and Pietro Ruggieri
Management of Displaced Midshaft Clavicle Fractures with Figure-of-Eight Bandage:
The Impact of Residual Shortening on Shoulder Function
Reprinted from: *J. Pers. Med.* **2022**, *12*, 759, doi:10.3390/jpm12050759 . . . . **103**

Claire Stark, John Cunningham, Peter Turner, Michael A. Johnson and Henrik C. Bäcker
App-Based Rehabilitation in Back Pain, a Systematic Review
Reprinted from: *J. Pers. Med.* **2022**, *12*, 1558, doi:10.3390/jpm12101558 . . . . **117**

Henrik Constantin Bäcker, Chia H. Wu, Dominik Pförringer, Wolf Petersen, Ulrich Stöckle
and Karl F. Braun
A Review of Functional Outcomes after the App-Based Rehabilitation of Patients with TKA and
THA
Reprinted from: *J. Pers. Med.* **2022**, *12*, 1342, doi:10.3390/jpm12081342 . . . . **126**

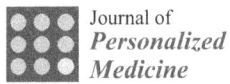

Article

Sterile Silicone Ring Tourniquets in Limb Surgery: A Prospective Clinical Trial in Pediatric Patients Undergoing Orthopedic Surgery

Kunhyung Bae [1], Gisu Kim [2], Amaal M. Aldosari [2,3], Yeonji Gim [2,4] and Yoon Hae Kwak [2,*]

1 Department of Orthopedic Surgery, Hanyang University Hospital, Hanyang University College of Medicine, 222 Wangsimni-ro, Seongdong-gu, Seoul 04763, Republic of Korea; bae_k_h@naver.com
2 Department of Orthopedic Surgery, Asan Medical Center Children's Hospital, University of Ulsan College of Medicine, 88, Olympic-ro, 43-gil, Songpa-gu, Seoul 05505, Republic of Korea; rlarl9744@naver.com (G.K.); dr_amaal@hotmail.com (A.M.A.); yeonji520@naver.com (Y.G.)
3 Department of Orthopaedic Surgery, Al Noor Specialist Hospital, Makkah 24242, Saudi Arabia
4 Department of Orthopaedic Surgery, Severance Hospital, Yonsei University College of Medicine, 50-1 Yonsei-ro, Seodaemoon-gu, Seoul 03722, Republic of Korea
* Correspondence: y.h.kwak@amc.seoul.kr; Tel.: +82-2-3010-3536

Abstract: Sterile silicone ring tourniquets (SSRTs) reduce intraoperative bleeding and provide a wide surgical view. Moreover, they reduce the risk of contamination and are cheaper than conventional pneumatic tourniquets. Our study describes the perioperative outcomes of sterile silicone ring tourniquet placement in pediatric patients undergoing orthopedic surgery. We prospectively recruited 27 pediatric patients aged < 18 years who underwent 30 orthopedic surgeries between March and September 2021. Following complete surgical draping, all operations were initiated by placing SSRTs. We investigated the demographic and clinical characteristics of these patients, details of the tourniquet used, and intra- and postoperative outcomes of tourniquet placement. Owing to the narrowness of tourniquet bands and tourniquet placement at the proximal ends of the extremities, wide surgical fields were achieved, without limiting joint range of motion. Bleeding control was effective. Tourniquets were applied and removed rapidly and safely, regardless of limb circumference. None of the patients experienced postoperative pain, paresthesia, skin problems at the application site, surgical site infections, ischemic problems, or deep vein thrombosis. SSRTs effectively reduced intraoperative blood loss and facilitated wide operative fields in pediatric patients with various limb sizes. These tourniquets allow quick, safe, and effective orthopedic surgery for pediatric patients.

Keywords: sterile silicone ring tourniquet; pediatric orthopedics; extremity surgery; bleeding control

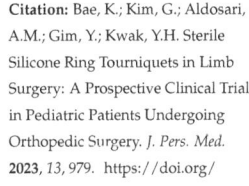

Citation: Bae, K.; Kim, G.; Aldosari, A.M.; Gim, Y.; Kwak, Y.H. Sterile Silicone Ring Tourniquets in Limb Surgery: A Prospective Clinical Trial in Pediatric Patients Undergoing Orthopedic Surgery. J. Pers. Med. 2023, 13, 979. https://doi.org/10.3390/jpm13060979

Academic Editors: Arne Kienzle and Henrik Bäcker

Received: 12 April 2023
Revised: 6 June 2023
Accepted: 7 June 2023
Published: 10 June 2023

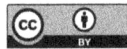

Copyright: © 2023 by the authors. Licensee MDPI, Basel, Switzerland. This article is an open access article distributed under the terms and conditions of the Creative Commons Attribution (CC BY) license (https://creativecommons.org/licenses/by/4.0/).

1. Introduction

Tourniquet use in orthopedic surgery enables bloodless operations, and facilitates the identification of important anatomical structures while also decreasing the anesthetic and operation time. However, the tourniquet itself is related to various complications such as skin and nerve injury, rhabdomyolysis, deep vein thrombosis, or compartment syndrome. Accordingly, many types of tourniquet systems have been invented and used by surgeon's preferences.

Conventional pneumatic tourniquets have been shown to control blood flow and reperfusion during surgical procedures effectively; moreover, their reusability also makes them economical [1]. Despite these advantages, there is a demand for other types of tourniquets in pediatric patients undergoing orthopedic surgery. Pneumatic tourniquet cuffs are relatively wide enough to block blood flow. As children have relatively short limbs, the wide cuffs of pneumatic tourniquets cover greater areas in children than in adults. This can be a major obstacle, especially in proximal limb surgery, because it might block the sight of the surgeon's field of view [2]. Additionally, the short limbs of infants and toddlers have a conical shape at the thigh, which often results in unintentional cuff sliding events and causes loss of arterial blood occlusion. Moreover, because limb size and circumference vary according to age, it is difficult to determine the adequate cuff size and amount of pressure to apply in pediatric patients. In addition, the skin and soft tissues are more delicate in children than in adults, increasing the probability of skin injury or chemical burns in the areas where the tourniquet was applied [3]. Furthermore, there is an issue of contamination of the tourniquet cuff; it can be a potential source of microbial colonization and may increase the surgical infection rate.

Owing to these drawbacks, Esmarch bandage tourniquets have been regarded as alternatives to conventional pneumatic tourniquets. They are also reusable, easy to sterilize, and allow blood exsanguination regardless of the limb circumference of the patients. However, Esmarch bandages still have wide cuffs, making it difficult to control the amount of pressure at the application site which can cause soft tissue damage [4].

Therefore, sterile silicone ring tourniquets have been suggested as good alternatives to pneumatic tourniquets. These tourniquets have only 2 cm wide cuffs, provide even pressure at compression sites, and can be applied in aseptic conditions [5]. Additionally, because it can be located at a more proximal site, we can achieve a wider surgical field without the risk of contamination. Although sterile silicone ring tourniquets have been frequently used and their outcomes have been reported in adult patients, only a few retrospective studies have evaluated their effects in pediatric patients [2,6].

This study aimed to investigate the effectiveness of sterile silicone ring tourniquets in pediatric patients undergoing orthopedic limb surgery. Both intraoperative and postoperative outcomes of sterile silicone ring tourniquet application and complications in pediatric patients undergoing orthopedic limb surgery were prospectively evaluated. We hypothesized that silicone ring tourniquets can work successfully in pediatric patients without perioperative complications.

2. Materials and Methods

2.1. Patient Selection

This study was approved by the Severance Hospital institutional review board (IRB No. 1-2020-0076). Patients who visited our pediatric orthopedic clinic between March 1st and September 30th, 2021 were prospectively recruited. Informed consent was obtained from all enrolled patients and their parents. Patients were included if they were (1) aged < 18 years and (2) scheduled to undergo upper or lower extremity in pediatric orthopedic surgery. Patients were excluded if the (1) expected tourniquet time was more than 2 h, (2) had poor skin condition where tourniquet would be applied, (3) were undergoing hip or shoulder joint surgery, (4) had unstable limb fractures, or (5) had musculoskeletal infections. Finally, a total of 27 patients (14 male, 13 female with 30 limbs) were included in the analysis.

2.2. Application of Sterile Silicone Ring Tourniquet in Limb Surgery

All surgeries in this study were performed by a single senior pediatric orthopedic surgeon (YHK). Sterile silicone ring tourniquets (Rapband®; Rapmedicare, Gyeonggi-do, Republic of Korea) (Figure 1) are designed for specific limb circumferences to provide preset pressure; unlike conventional pneumatic tourniquets, which allow the operator to control the applied pressure. They applied to provide different pressures with 4 sizes; small, medium, large, and extra-large sterile silicone ring tourniquets respectively providing pressures of 200 ± 20, 230 ± 40, 310 ± 40, and 320 ± 20 mmHg. The sizes were categorized by patient limb circumference, the small model was fit for 14 to 21 cm, the medium was 22 to 39 cm, the large was 40 to 54 cm, and the extra-large was more than 54 cm. Each tourniquet comprised a sterile silicone ring wrapped in a stockinet and two pulled straps. After complete aseptic draping, the most appropriately sized sterile silicone ring tourniquet was selected after measuring the limb circumference of the occlusion site with sterile tape measure. After an approximate ring tourniquet was selected, it was applied to the limb. The tourniquet was placed on the distal part of the limb and the two straps were pulled to the proximal part of the limb. The sterile silicone ring was unrolled to its final location at the proximal site with exsanguination of the remaining blood. The final width of the cuff after application was 2 to 3 cm. After the main surgical procedures were completed, the tourniquet was removed using a blade or pair of scissors.

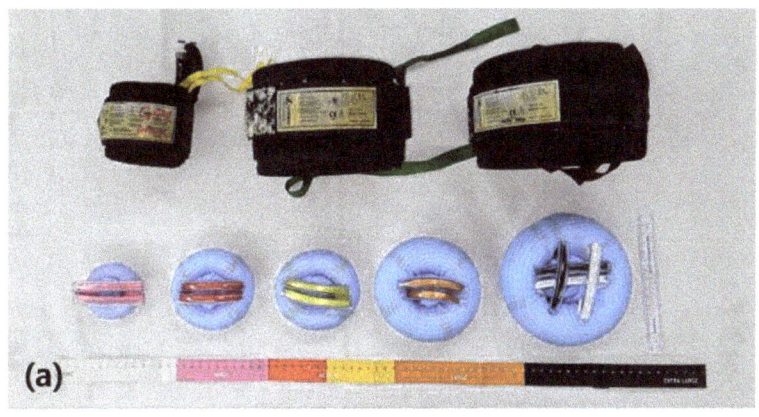

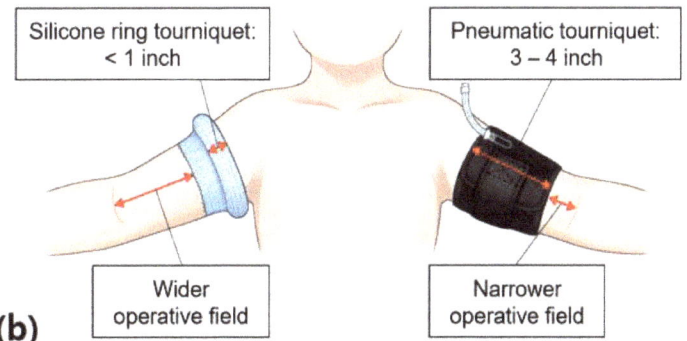

Figure 1. (a) Sterile silicone ring tourniquet and conventional pneumatic tourniquet, and (b) detailed illustration of applied states.

2.3. Investigated Variables and Statistical Analysis

We recorded patient demographic characteristics and tourniquet information, including age, sex, diagnosis, surgical procedure, laterality, tourniquet application area, limb circumference, tourniquet size, and application time. Tourniquet outcomes were grouped as intraoperative and postoperative outcomes. The intraoperative outcomes included tourniquet application and removal times, changes in elbow or knee joint range of motion (ROM) before and after tourniquet application, adequate operative field visualization, and bleeding control evaluated by the number of gauze pads used. Postoperative outcomes included skin condition at the application site, surgical site infection, ischemic complications (compartment syndrome and distal neurovascular compromise), and deep vein thrombosis. For the patients aged > 5 years, pain and paresthesia at the tourniquet site were evaluated 24 h after surgery. The pain was evaluated by a numerical rating scale (NRS), a pain screening tool which rates the pain from 0 (no pain) to 10 (worst pain). Statistical analyses were performed using Microsoft Excel 2010 (Microsoft, Redmond, WA, USA).

3. Results

The demographic characteristics of the patients and tourniquet information are presented in Table 1. The mean patient age was 9.8 ± 5.3 years (range: 1 to 17 years) and the mean limb circumference at the application site was 35.9 ± 16.1 cm (range: 15 to 65 cm). Following the manufacturer's guide, all four sizes of tourniquets were used for operation in this study. All included operations were completed within 2 h of tourniquet application, with a mean operation time of 36.5 ± 29.7 min (range: 5 to 110 min). The types of operations performed were various; fracture reductions, soft tissue surgeries, deformity correction, and implant removal.

Table 1. Demographic and clinical characteristics of the patients and information of applied silicone ring tourniquets in this study.

Patient No.	Case no.	Age (year)	Sex	Diagnosis	Operation Procedure	Laterality	Application Area	Circumference [1] (cm)	Time (min)	Size
1	1	3	F	Congenital trigger thumb	A1 pulley release	R	Upper arm	17	11	S
2	2	4	M	Congenital trigger thumb	A1 pulley release	R	Upper arm	20	10	S
3	3	10	F	Pilomatrichoma	Mass excision	L	Upper arm	27	19	M
4	4	10	F	Ganglion cyst	Mass excision	R	Thigh	45	47	L
5	5	17	F	Lower leg deformity due to neonatal sepsis	Plate change	R	Thigh	50	73	L
	6			Lower leg deformity due to neonatal sepsis	Plate change	L	Thigh	48	51	L
6	7	12	F	Talocalcaneal coalition	Coalition resection	R	Thigh	49	59	L
7	8	15	F	Jones fracture	ORIF by screw	R	Thigh	58	31	XL
8	9	7	M	Both forearm fracture	CRIF with flexible elastic nail	L	Upper arm	23	21	M
9	10	14	M	Distal femur hemiepiphysiodesis status	Implant removal	L	Thigh	44	9	L
10	11	9	M	Femur shaft fracture fixation status	Implant removal	L	Thigh	37	48	M
11	12	14	F	Accessory navicular bone	Accessory bone resection	R	Thigh	47	12	L
12	13	17	F	Distal tibia fracture fixation status	Implant removal	L	Thigh	50	32	L
13	14	11	M	Trevor's disease	Mass excision	R	Upper arm	23	29	M
14	15	16	F	4th toe epidermoid cyst	Mass excision	R	Thigh	60	26	X
15	16	4	M	Congenital trigger thumb	A1 pulley release	R	Upper arm	18	8	S
	17			Congenital trigger thumb	A1 pulley release	L	Upper arm	19	7	S
16	18	3	M	Congenital trigger thumb	A1 pulley release	L	Upper arm	18	7	S
17	19	1	M	Congenital trigger thumb	A1 pulley release	L	Upper arm	15	10	S
18	20	5	M	Congenital trigger thumb	A1 pulley release	L	Upper arm	23	12	M
19	21	5	M	Lateral condylar fracture fixation status	Implant removal	L	Upper arm	24	90	M
20	22	16	M	Distal femur fracture fixation status	Implant removal	L	Thigh	65	110	XL
21	23	12	M	Distal femur hemiepiphysiodesis status due to idiopathic genu valgum	Implant removal	R	Thigh	46	40	L

Table 1. Cont.

Patient No.	Case no.	Age (year)	Sex	Diagnosis	Operation Procedure	Laterality	Application Area	Circumference[1] (cm)	Time (min)	Size
	24			Distal femur hemiepiphysiodesis status due to idiopathic genu valgum	Implant removal	L	Thigh	45	35	L
22	25	1	M	Hand preaxial polydactyly	Extra digit excision	R	Upper arm	15	80	S
23	26	12	F	Revisional Achilles tendon Z plasty	CMT with Achilles tightness	L	Thigh	43	85	L
24	27	4	F	Congenital trigger thumb	A1 pulley release	R	Thigh	17	5	S
25	28	12	M	Fifth finger proximal phalanx malunion	Deformity correction by pinning	R	Thigh	23	80	M
26	29	17	F	Lateral malleolar fracture fixation status	Implant removal	L	Thigh	47	35	L
27	30	14	F	Achilles tightness	Achilles Tendon lengthening	R	Thigh	60	12	XL

no, number; cm, centimeter; min, minute; M, male; F, female; R, right; L, left; S, small; M, medium; L, large; XL, extra-large; ORIF, open reduction and internal fixation; CRIF, close reduction and internal fixation; CMT, Charcot-Marie-Tooth disease. [1] Circumference at the tourniquet application area.

The perioperative tourniquet outcomes are presented in Table 2. All tourniquets were applied and removed within 15 s in the operative field. Knee or elbow joint ROM was the same before and after the tourniquet application. Therefore, there were no postural limitations during surgery (Figure 2).

Table 2. Intraoperative and postoperative outcomes of sterile silicone ring tourniquets.

Tourniquet Outcome Parameters	Results
Intraoperative Outcome	
Tourniquet application time (s)	Mean: 7.5 ± 2.8 (range: 4 to 15)
Tourniquet removal time (s)	Mean: 5.4 ± 1.4 (range: 4 to 10)
Joint ROM between pre- and post-tourniquet application [1]	All cases showed the same joint ROM after the tourniquet application
Operative field visualization	All cases had a sufficient operative field for surgery even after applying a tourniquet
Bleeding control (by gauze counting)	Gauze not used to control bleeding in 27 cases Two cases used one piece of gauze—ORIF by screw for Jones fracture, mass excision for Trevor's disease One case used two pieces of gauze—Plate change for deformity due to neonatal sepsis
Postoperative outcome	
Skin problem at the tourniquet application site	None of these cases experienced skin problems, including bullae, necrosis, hematoma, contusion, or burn
Surgical site infection	None of these cases experienced surgical site infection after follow-up periods
Ischemic complications	None of these cases showed ischemic complications, including compartment syndrome or neuromuscular compromise
Deep vein thrombosis	None of these cases showed deep vein thrombosis
Pain at tourniquet application site [2]	All 18 patients aged >5 years reported an NRS score of 0
Abnormal sensory change at tourniquet application site [2]	None of the 18 patients aged >5 years experienced abnormal sensory changes

sec, second; ROM, range of motion; ORIF, open reduction, and internal fixation; NRS, numerical rating scale. [1] The elbow joint was evaluated for upper extremity surgeries, and the knee joint was evaluated for lower extremity surgeries. [2] Evaluated 24 h after surgery in patients aged ≥5 years.

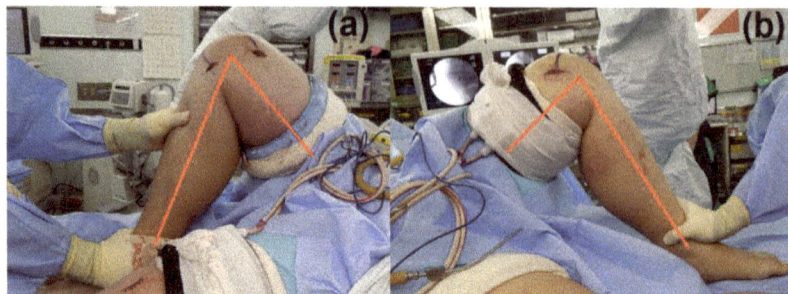

Figure 2. Knee joint range of motion (ROM) between sterile silicone ring and pneumatic tourniquets. Comparison of knee joint range of motion (ROM) between sterile silicone ring tourniquet in the right lower leg (**a**) and pneumatic compression tourniquet (**b**) in the left leg for a 12-year-old male patient with both side hemiepiphysiodesis. After the sterile silicone ring tourniquet application, the right knee joint still had full flexion with a wide operative field; however, the left knee joint showed limited flexion due to the inflated pneumatic cuff and narrow operative field.

The thin width of the sterile ring tourniquet made it possible to easily expose lesions in the proximal limb, as it provided a sufficient surgical field (Figure 3). For the aspect of bleeding control, the need for intraoperative gauze usage was only observed in 3 surgeries, and the other 27 surgeries did not need gauze to stop bleeding.

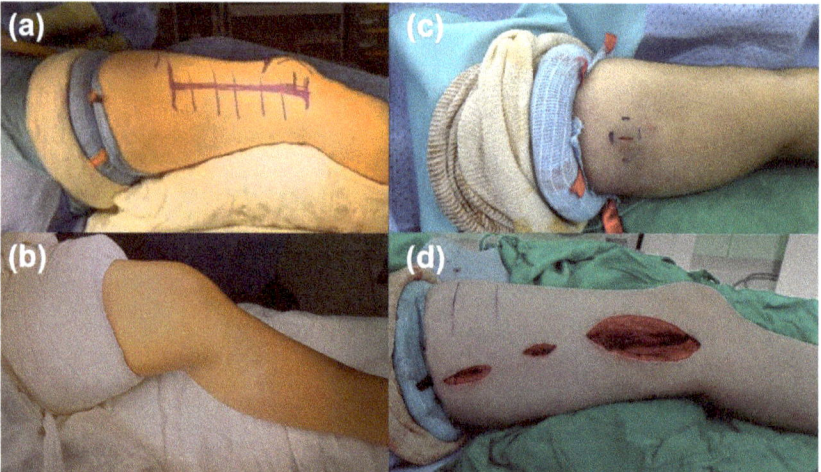

Figure 3. Size of surgical fields between sterile silicone ring and pneumatic tourniquets. Comparison of surgical fields for (**a**) a sterile silicone ring tourniquet and (**b**) a conventional pneumatic tourniquet. Sterile silicone ring tourniquet cuff is much narrower than conventional pneumatic tourniquet cuff (2 to 3 cm vs. 8 to 16 cm, which allows for better surgical site exposure for proximal thigh lesions. Surgical field after application of a sterile silicone ring tourniquet in (**c**) a 10-year-old girl with pilomatricoma excision at the upper right arm and (**d**) a 16-year-old boy with open reduction and internal fixation of a femur shaft fracture. Both patients required maximal exposure of the proximal limb, making it mandatory to use sterile silicone ring tourniquets rather than pneumatic tourniquets.

The postoperative evaluation showed there was no soft tissue damage, such as skin necrosis, abrasion, and bullae in all patients (Figure 4). There was no surgical site infection during follow-up periods. None of the patients experienced major problems such as compartment syndrome, deep vein thrombosis, or distal neurovascular compromise due to ischemic damage to the tourniquet. All patients aged ≥5 years reported there was no pain (NRS score 0) and neurological deficits around the tourniquet ring site 24 h after surgery.

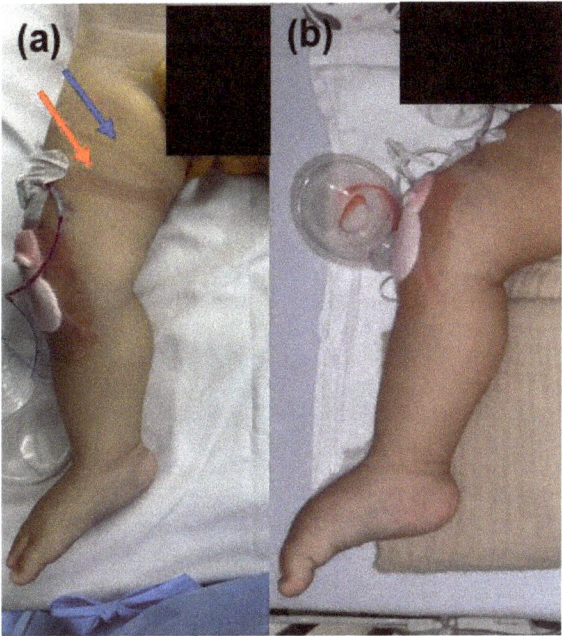

Figure 4. The reversible compression effect of the sterile silicone ring on the skin. (**a**) Compressed skin mark (red arrow) immediately after sterile silicone ring tourniquet removal. However, there was no bullae, blister, or hematoma. Blue arrow shows the marks on the skin after U-drape (**b**) Compressed skin lesion by silicone ring returned to a normal status 8 h after silicone ring tourniquet removal.

4. Discussion

The sterile silicone ring tourniquet is a single-use device that enables the exposure of a larger proximal area compared to conventional pneumatic compression tourniquets. We conducted a prospective study on the perioperative outcome of a sterile silicone ring tourniquet for limb surgery with a circumference of 15 cm to 65 cm for patients aged 1 to 17 years. It was easily applicable and removable in the operation field. The volume of the sterile silicone ring tourniquet was small and did not restrict joint movement during surgery. The postoperative evaluation showed no evidence of surgical site infections, skin problems, ischemic changes, or any abnormal symptoms when the tourniquet application was completed within 2 h. This study found that sterile silicone ring tourniquets were also effective and safe in pediatric patients with varying limb sizes and circumferences.

4.1. Sterile Silicone Ring Tourniquets for Pediatric Patients

Limb circumference increases as children grow until they reach skeletal maturity [7,8]. Therefore, it is essential to select appropriate tourniquet cuffs and pressure based on the circumference of individual limbs in pediatric patients undergoing orthopedic surgery. Because pneumatic tourniquet cuffs must be sterilized for intraoperative use, the cuff size must be determined at least several hours before surgery. In contrast, cuff sizes for silicone ring tourniquets can be determined based on limb circumference by tape measuring after surgical draping. Even for various limb circumferences, it is possible to use it immediately because there are sterilized single-use cuffs prepared. In addition, the nature of pediatric fractures, such as supracondylar and lateral condylar fractures, can lead to intraoperative changes from pre-planned surgical methods, including conversion from closed reduction to open reduction [9,10]. This conversion is difficult in the absence of a sterilized pneumatic tourniquet. In contrast, silicone ring tourniquets can always be applied, even during unplanned alterations of the surgical methods; moreover, both application and removal can be completed within 15 s. In pediatric trauma surgery where a possibility of surgical method conversion may be required, the silicone ring tourniquet presents several advantages over conventional pneumatic tourniquet.

4.2. Intraoperative Outcomes of Sterile Silicone Ring Tourniquet-Surgical Fields

Sufficient operative fields were secured in all 30 limbs analyzed in this study. Especially in the proximal site of upper arm or thigh operations, a silicone ring tourniquet enables the operator a wide view (Figure 2). The traditional pneumatic cuff was too wide to be used in upper arm or thigh operation, however, the proximal limb length exposed by ring-type tourniquets is longer than that exposed by conventional pneumatic tourniquets [11,12]. This is because pneumatic cuffs are 8 to 14 cm wide when added to surgical drapes, making it difficult to expose the proximal surgical site in young children with short limb lengths. In contrast, silicone ring tourniquets provide better limb exposure because the final cuff width is approximately 2 cm. This has been a great advantage in operations that require maximal exposure of the upper thigh or arm, such as soft tissue tumor removal or proximal limb fixation surgery [13]. In addition, the application of silicone ring tourniquets did not decrease joint ROM. In obese patients, the thickness of inflated pneumatic cuffs makes it difficult to obtain full ROM during surgery (Figure 3b). In contrast, because they are narrower, silicone ring tourniquets do not alter joint ROM even after application. These tourniquets are not restricted by changes in posture, thus allowing for an easier surgical approach. Moreover, bleeding control with silicone ring tourniquets was similar to that of conventional tourniquets in adults undergoing orthopedic surgery [14]. In this study, most operations were bloodless and gauze was generally not required. Only three cases required gauze for bleeding control, two cases one piece of gauze, and one case two pieces of gauze. Therefore, this type of tourniquet also effectively minimizes blood loss in pediatric orthopedic surgery. In addition, the application and removal time of sterile silicone ring tourniquet is 7.5 s and 5.4 s, respectively. It is a fast and easy way because one just needs to apply the tourniquet by rolling it from the distal to the proximal part and remove it to cut the tourniquet with a scalpel. In contrast, conventional tourniquet application is much more complex. The application involves tightening the cuff for a snug fit by pulling the straps and fasteners around the limb in opposite directions.

4.3. Postoperative Outcomes of Sterile Silicone Ring Tourniquet

None of the patients in the present study experienced skin problems such as bullae, necrosis, hematoma, contusion, or burn wounds at the tourniquet application site. Because children have softer and more fragile soft tissue than adults, tourniquets may be harmful postoperatively [2]. There are several reports of burns, abrasions, or hematomas at the application site with the pneumatic tourniquet, however, proper application of skin protection can protect the soft tissue from damage [3,15]. In this study, none of the patients experienced skin or soft tissue problems even 24 h postoperatively. Especially, there were 4 patients who were ≤3 years old who had more delicate soft tissues than older children. Therefore, even in toddlers, the silicone ring tourniquet would not cause soft tissue damage if used within proper operation time.

In addition, none of the patients experienced surgical site infection. Although the reuse of pneumatic tourniquets is economical, they can be a source of infection even after ethylene oxide sterilization [16]. Such equipment has the potential to colonize bacteria, increasing the possibility of transmitting pathogens to patients through the operating room. These surgical site infections increase the medical burden and consume medical resources, but also have harmful effects on the patients by repetitive blood tests, antibiotic usage, increasing length of hospitalization, and the possibility of reoperation [17]. There is one study reported that bacterial contamination in two-thirds of orthopedic surgical tourniquets with normal flora, such as coagulase-negative *Staphylococcus* spp., Staphylococcus aureus, suggesting that bacteria may be transferred between operated patients [18]. In contrast, silicone ring tourniquets are both sterile and disposable, thereby reducing the risk of surgical site infections [18].

Tourniquet use has also been associated with ischemic complications and deep vein thrombosis. High pressure and prolonged obstruction of arterial blood flow induce ischemic changes in the limbs. Moreover, ischemic tissue perfusion after blood circulation resumes can lead to secondary injury, including compartment syndrome and distal neurovascular problems, with the remaining blood possibly causing deep vein thrombosis [4,19]. Ischemic soft tissue damage did not differ between silicone rings and pneumatic tourniquets; therefore, customary tourniquet time within 2 h is safe for both types of tourniquets [20]. In addition, silicone ring tourniquets effectively minimize residual blood in the extremities by compressing the limb while unrolling it from the distal end to the proximal site. This procedure provides effective exsanguination and may significantly reduce deep vein thrombosis. Tourniquet pain originated from both compression effects of anatomical structures and ischemic changes; however, which etiologies have a main role is debatable. None of the patients in the present study experienced pain or sensory problems at the tourniquet site within 24 h postoperatively. According to previous studies, the incidence of pain and paresthesia among patients who underwent silicone ring tourniquet application was comparable to or lower than the incidence of these complications among patients who underwent pneumatic tourniquet application; its incidence is 1/50,000 and 1/5000, respectively [12,21,22]. Lee et al. recently reported in adult studies that 13.3% of patients felt higher pain in the pneumatic tourniquet, 76.7% of patients felt the same, and 10% of patients experienced higher pain in the silicon ring tourniquet-applied lower extremity [23]. However, pain associated with the use of tourniquets was first studied in 1952 and a number of mechanisms have been proposed as the cause. The exact etiology is unclear, but it is thought to be due to a cutaneous neural mechanism. The incidence of tourniquet pain was directly related to the duration of tourniquet use and was higher in cases with regional anesthesia [24]. The most important point was neurological compromise occurred in the silicone ring tourniquet with over 120 min of application time, over the recommended time. You should adhere to the principle of tourniquet use, including the time of application. There was one study that compared the pain score of pneumatic compression and silicone ring tourniquet in adult patients who underwent local anesthesia, the results of pain score and paresthesia were significantly lower in the silicone ring tourniquet group [23]. Moreover, considering that continuously publishing results show that the narrow silicone ring tourniquet causes less nerve damage, neurological problems are also safe for children who use the silicone ring tourniquet [24].

The present study has several limitations. First, it was a prospective clinical trial and not a comparative study. The target patient population was heterogeneous, with patients undergoing different parts of limbs with kinds of surgery. However, the strength of this study is its diversity of patients group of various ages and limb sizes, because it implies that silicone ring tourniquet has versatility in the pediatric orthopedic field. Even though these characteristics are in pediatric studies, further study should be considered for comparison with current widely used pneumatic tourniquets or Esmarch bandages. Second, this study reported the short-term results of sterile silicone ring tourniquet application. However, most complications associated with tourniquet application appear within a short period of time, suggesting that a short follow-up period may provide significant results; nevertheless, long-term follow-up results are warranted. Finally, the study had a limited sample size, with only 30 cases among 27 patients included. Because silicone ring tourniquets were developed for use in adults, only a few studies have evaluated these tourniquets in pediatric patients. Therefore, future comparative trials with a larger number of patients are warranted.

5. Conclusions

Sterile silicone ring tourniquets have easy and fast applications compared to preset pressure models. As opposed to concerns about pressure-focused narrow tourniquets, this study showed no pain, nerve symptoms, or skin problems in vulnerable pediatric patients. In addition, unlike conventional pneumatic tourniquets or Esmarch bandages, SSRTs apply uniform pressure to the limb during the application, reducing the risk of deep vein thrombosis. These tourniquets provide a sufficient surgical field in pediatric patients undergoing orthopedic surgery on their extremities because they are located at a more proximal site on the extremities with narrow cuff width. Moreover, their application within 2 h can ensure successful bleeding control without soft tissue complications, neurovascular compression, or surgical site infection.

Author Contributions: Conceptualization: Y.H.K.; methodology: K.B., G.K., A.M.A., Y.G. and Y.H.K.; formal analysis and investigation: K.B., G.K., A.M.A., Y.G. and Y.H.K.; writing—original draft preparation: K.B., G.K. and Y.H.K.; writing—review and editing: K.B. and Y.H.K.; funding acquisition: Y.H.K.; supervision: Y.H.K. All authors have read and agreed to the published version of the manuscript.

Funding: This research was funded by Rapmedicare Co., Ltd., Republic of Korea.

Institutional Review Board Statement: The study was conducted according to the guidelines of the Declaration of Helsinki, and approved by the Institutional Review Board of Severance hospital (IRB No. 1-2020-0076 21 December 2020).

Informed Consent Statement: Informed consent was obtained from all subjects involved in the study or their parents.

Data Availability Statement: The datasets used and analyzed during the current study are available from the corresponding author on reasonable request.

Acknowledgments: The authors would like to thank the Asan Medical Contents Unit for artistic support related to this work.

Conflicts of Interest: The funders had no role in the design of the study; in the collection, analyses, or interpretation of data; in the writing of the manuscript; or in the decision to publish the results.

References

1. Fitzgibbons, P.G.; Digiovanni, C.; Hares, S.; Akelman, E. Safe tourniquet use: A review of the evidence. *J. Am. Acad. Orthop. Surg.* **2012**, *20*, 310–319. [CrossRef]
2. Eidelman, M.; Katzman, A.; Bialik, V. A novel elastic exsanguination tourniquet as an alternative to the pneumatic cuff in pediatric orthopedic limb surgery. *J. Pediatr. Orthop. B* **2006**, *15*, 379–384. [CrossRef]
3. Tredwell, S.J.; Wilmink, M.; Inkpen, K.; McEwen, J.A. Pediatric tourniquets: Analysis of cuff and limb interface, current practice, and guidelines for use. *J. Pediatr. Orthop.* **2001**, *21*, 671–676. [CrossRef] [PubMed]
4. Abraham, E.; Amirouche, F.M. Pressure controlled Esmarch bandage used as a tourniquet. *Foot. Ankle. Int.* **2000**, *21*, 686–689. [CrossRef] [PubMed]
5. Bourquelot, P.; Levy, B.I. Narrow elastic disposable tourniquet (Hemaclear®) vs. traditional wide pneumatic tourniquet for creation or revision of hemodialysis angioaccesses. *J. Vasc. Access.* **2016**, *17*, 205–209. [CrossRef]
6. Franzone, J.M.; Yang, J.H.; Herzenberg, J.E. Reuse of single-use HemaClear exsanguination tourniquets: A technique note. *J. Long. Term Eff. Med. Implants* **2017**, *27*, 59–65. [CrossRef]
7. Mramba, L.; Ngari, M.; Mwangome, M.; Muchai, L.; Bauni, E.; Walker, A.S.; Gibb, D.N.; Fegan, G.; Berkley, J.A. A growth reference for mid upper arm circumference for age among school age children and adolescents, and validation for mortality: Growth curve construction and longitudinal cohort study. *BMJ* **2017**, *358*, j3423. [CrossRef]
8. Saeed, W.; Akbar, A.; Waseem, M.; Kuchinski, A.M.; Xu, H.; Gibson, R.W. Addition of midthigh circumference improves predictive ability of Broselow tape weight estimation. *Pediatr. Emerg. Care* **2022**, *38*, 448–452. [CrossRef]
9. Latario, L.D.; Lubitz, M.G.; Narain, A.S.; Swart, E.F.; Mortimer, E.S. Which pediatric supracondylar humerus fractures are high risk for conversion to open reduction? *J. Pediatr. Orthop. B* **2022**. [CrossRef]
10. Kang, M.S.; Alfadhil, R.A.; Park, S.S. Outcomes of arthroscopy-assisted closed reduction and percutaneous pinning for a displaced pediatric lateral condylar humeral fracture. *J. Pediatr. Orthop.* **2019**, *39*, 548–551. [CrossRef]
11. Drosos, G.I.; Stavropoulos, N.I.; Kazakos, K.; Tripsianis, G.; Ververidis, A.; Verettas, D.A. Silicone ring versus pneumatic cuff tourniquet: A comparative quantitative study in healthy individuals. *Arch. Orthop. Trauma Surg.* **2011**, *131*, 447–454. [CrossRef]

12. Park, K.K.; Cho, B.W.; Lee, W.S.; Kwon, H.M. Silicone ring tourniquet could be a substitute for a conventional tourniquet in total knee arthroplasty with a longer surgical field: A prospective comparative study in simultaneous total knee arthroplasty. *BMC Musculoskelet. Disord.* **2023**, *24*, 363.
13. Ehlinger, M.; Adam, P.; Abane, L.; Arlettaz, Y.; Bonnomet, F. Minimally-invasive internal fixation of extra-articular distal femur fractures using a locking plate: Tricks of the trade. *Orthop. Traumatol. Surg. Res.* **2011**, *97*, 201–205. [CrossRef]
14. Brin, Y.S.; Feldman, V.; Ron, G.I.; Markushevitch, M.; Regev, A.; Stern, A. The Sterile Elastic Exsanguination Tourniquet vs. the Pneumatic Tourniquet for total knee arthroplasty. *J. Arthroplast.* **2015**, *30*, 595–599. [CrossRef] [PubMed]
15. Noordin, S.; McEwen, J.A.; Kragh, J.F., Jr.; Eisen, A.; Masri, B.A. Surgical tourniquets in orthopaedics. *J. Bone Jt. Surg. Am.* **2009**, *91*, 2958–2967. [CrossRef] [PubMed]
16. Mufarrih, S.H.; Qureshi, N.Q.; Rashid, R.H.; Ahmed, B.; Irfan, S.; Zubairi, A.J.; Noordin, S. Microbial colonization of pneumatic tourniquets in the orthopedic operating room. *Cureus* **2019**, *11*, e5308. [CrossRef] [PubMed]
17. Brennan, S.A.; Walls, R.J.; Smyth, E.; Al Mulla, T.; O'Byrne, J.M. Tourniquets and exsanguinators: A potential source of infection in the orthopedic operating theater? *Acta Orthop.* **2009**, *80*, 251–255. [CrossRef]
18. Thompson, S.M.; Middleton, M.; Farook, M.; Cameron-Smith, A.; Bone, S.; Hassan, A. The effect of sterile versus non-sterile tourniquets on microbiological colonisation in lower limb surgery. *Ann. R. Coll. Surg. Engl.* **2011**, *93*, 589–590. [CrossRef]
19. Xie, J.; Yu, H.; Wang, F.; Jing, J.; Li, J. A comparison of thrombosis in total knee arthroplasty with and without a tourniquet: A meta-analysis of randomized controlled trials. *J. Orthop. Surg. Res.* **2021**, *16*, 408. [CrossRef]
20. León-Muñoz, V.J.; Lisón-Almagro, A.J.; Hernández-García, C.H.; López-López, M. Silicone ring tourniquet versus pneumatic cuff tourniquet in total knee arthroplasty surgery: A randomised comparative study. *J. Orthop.* **2018**, *15*, 545–548. [CrossRef]
21. Kamath, K.; Kamath, S.U.; Tejaswi, P. Incidence and factors influencing tourniquet pain. *Chin. J. Traumatol.* **2021**, *24*, 291–294. [CrossRef] [PubMed]
22. Drosos, G.I.; Kiziridis, G.; Aggelopoulou, C.; Galiatsatos, D.; Anastassopoulos, G.; Ververidis, A.; Kazakos, K. The effect of the silicone ring tourniquet and standard pneumatic tourniquet on the motor nerve conduction, pain and grip strength in healthy volunteers. *Arch. Bone Jt. Surg.* **2016**, *4*, 16–22. [PubMed]
23. Mohan, A.; Baskaradas, A.; Solan, M.; Magnussen, P. Pain and paraesthesia produced by silicone ring and pneumatic tourniquets. *J. Hand Surg. Eur.* **2011**, *36*, 215–218. [CrossRef] [PubMed]
24. Weatherholt, A.M.; VanWye, W.R.; Lohmann, J.; Owens, J.G. The effect of cuff width for determining limb occlusion pressure: A comparison of blood flow restriction devices. *Int. J. Exerc. Sci.* **2019**, *12*, 136–143. [PubMed]

Disclaimer/Publisher's Note: The statements, opinions and data contained in all publications are solely those of the individual author(s) and contributor(s) and not of MDPI and/or the editor(s). MDPI and/or the editor(s) disclaim responsibility for any injury to people or property resulting from any ideas, methods, instructions or products referred to in the content.

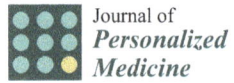

Article

Comparing the 30-Day Mortality for Hip Fractures in Patients with and without COVID-19: An Updated Meta-Analysis

Sojune Hwang, Chiwon Ahn * and Moonho Won

Department of Emergency Medicine, College of Medicine, Chung-Ang University, Seoul 06974, Republic of Korea; junee327@cauhs.or.kr (S.H.); wonmh0922@cauhs.or.kr (M.W.)
* Correspondence: cahn@cau.ac.kr

Abstract: We conducted an updated meta-analysis to evaluate the 30-day mortality of hip fractures during the COVID-19 pandemic and assess mortality rates by country. We systematically searched Medline, EMBASE, and the Cochrane Library up to November 2022 for studies on the 30-day mortality of hip fractures during the pandemic. Two reviewers used the Newcastle–Ottawa tool to independently assess the methodological quality of the included studies. We conducted a meta-analysis and systematic review including 40 eligible studies with 17,753 patients with hip fractures, including 2280 patients with COVID-19 (12.8%). The overall 30-day mortality rate for hip fractures during the pandemic was 12.6% from published studies. The 30-day mortality of patients with hip fractures who had COVID-19 was significantly higher than those without COVID-19 (OR, 7.10; 95% CI, 5.51–9.15; I^2 = 57%). The hip fracture mortality rate increased during the pandemic and varied by country, with the highest rates found in Europe, particularly the United Kingdom (UK) and Spain. COVID-19 may have contributed to the increased 30-day mortality rate in hip fracture patients. The mortality rate of hip fracture in patients without COVID-19 did not change during the pandemic.

Keywords: hip fracture; COVID-19; pandemic; mortality

Citation: Hwang, S.; Ahn, C.; Won, M. Comparing the 30-Day Mortality for Hip Fractures in Patients with and without COVID-19: An Updated Meta-Analysis. *J. Pers. Med.* **2023**, *13*, 669. https://doi.org/10.3390/jpm13040669

Academic Editors: Arne Kienzle and Henrik Bäcker

Received: 18 February 2023
Revised: 4 April 2023
Accepted: 13 April 2023
Published: 15 April 2023

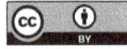

Copyright: © 2023 by the authors. Licensee MDPI, Basel, Switzerland. This article is an open access article distributed under the terms and conditions of the Creative Commons Attribution (CC BY) license (https://creativecommons.org/licenses/by/4.0/).

1. Introduction

The COVID-19 pandemic has significantly impacted the healthcare system and redirected many of its resources [1]. There was a shortage of information about the disease, and many healthcare systems faced collapse in the early stages of the pandemic [2–4]. This caused a gap in care for non-COVID-19 diseases, including delays in diagnosis and treatment due to additional screening processes in hospitals and emergency care systems [5]. The pandemic also impacted emergency medical services for diseases such as acute myocardial infarction, stroke, out-of-hospital cardiac arrest, and sepsis [3,4,6–9]. During the pandemic, the epidemiological characteristics of known diseases have also changed. In fact, for out-of-hospital cardiac arrest, there was an increase in arrests occurring at home and a decrease in the frequency of shockable rhythms. These changes were associated with an increase in out-of-hospital cardiac arrest cases and longer transport times to hospitals following COVID infection [8,9]. Furthermore, various surgical diseases have either contributed to the increase in the frequency of surgical decisions during the pandemic or led to a rise in complications due to delays in surgery. For example, patients with appendicitis faced delays in surgery and increased complications [10]. Social distancing and self-isolation measures during the pandemic further exacerbated these issues.

Hip fractures, a growing public health concern among the elderly, have high mortality rates [11]. Hip fracture management indicates the quality of care for elderly patients and how trauma services are functioning [12]. Despite the decreased number of trauma patients due to reduced activity during the pandemic, the number of hip fractures in elderly individuals was unchanged [13]. The social distancing, self-isolation, and limited public medical services during the pandemic made caring for the elderly more difficult.

COVID-19 screening processes may delay surgery for patients with hip fractures [14]. The pandemic also increases the risk of death for those with hip fractures, with previous meta-analyses reporting higher mortality rates for patients with both hip fractures and COVID-19 compared to those with hip fractures alone [15,16].

These meta-analyses evaluated the effect of COVID-19 infection on the outcomes for patients with hip fractures and showed significant results. Even after that, numerous studies investigated the effect of COVID-19 on the outcomes of hip fracture. At this point, we needed to analyze the changed results compared to the results of previous studies. Therefore, we conducted an updated meta-analysis on the 30-day mortality of hip fractures for individuals with and without COVID-19 and also analyzed the 30-day mortality of hip fractures during the pandemic based on published cases.

2. Materials and Methods

2.1. Reporting Guidelines and Protocol Registration

This study complied with the Preferred Reporting Items for Systematic Reviews and Meta-analyses and the Meta-analysis of Observational Studies in Epidemiology Guidelines for Reporting Information from Observational Studies [17,18]. We prospectively registered with the PROSPERO registry (CRD42022385443).

2.2. Eligibility Criteria

We applied the Population, Intervention, Comparison, and Outcome (PICO) clinical question. We performed a literature search and selected eligible studies. The study outcomes were then evaluated in a meta-analysis. The PICO questions were as follows: population (P) = all adult patients with hip fractures visiting the emergency room regardless conduction of operation; exposure (I) = COVID-19 infection; comparator (C) = non-infection; outcome (O) = 30-day mortality.

2.3. Search Strategy

Two reviewers systematically searched several electronic databases (Medline via OVID interface, Embase, and Cochrane Library) for studies on the outcomes of adult hip fracture patients with COVID-19 infection compared to those with no infection. The search terms were "Coronavirus" or "COVID-19" or "SARS-CoV" or "2019-nCoV" or "Severe Acute Respiratory Syndrome", and "Hip Fractures" or "Femoral Fractures" or "femoral shaft" or "femur shaft" or "periprosthetic" or "femur neck" or "trochanteric" or "intracapsular". We summarize the detailed search strategy for each database in Supplementary Table S1.

2.4. Study Selection

Two reviewers independently screened the title, abstract, and type of each identified article, excluding irrelevant studies. First, we eliminated duplicate studies in which the titles, authors, and publication years were the same. We then excluded all reviews, case reports, case series, editorials, comments, or meta-analyses; animal studies; research with irrelevant study populations; and those with inappropriate controls. A third reviewer intervened if the two reviewers disagreed about a study, and differences were discussed until a consensus was achieved. Finally, we included studies that evaluated the outcomes of patients with hip fractures during the COVID-19 pandemic and compared them to those reported before the pandemic and studies on adult populations over 18 years of age. We also excluded studies that (1) included patients aged less than 18 years, (2) provided no comparisons or outcomes, and (3) were non-original articles. In addition, we included fracture patients with or without surgery. We subsequently reviewed the full text of potentially relevant articles that met the inclusion criteria.2.5. Data Extraction

The two reviewers independently extracted the following information from the included studies: (1) publication details (author and year), (2) study type and settings, (3) patient population (region, number of participating center(s), number of patients, and patient demographics and comorbidities), (4) the rate of operation, (5) the length of hospital stay, and (6) 30-day mortality. Discrepancies between reviewers were resolved by consensus.

2.5. Quality Assessment in Individual Studies

We assessed the risk of bias in each study with the Newcastle–Ottawa Quality Assessment for Cohort Studies tool [19]. Each study was assigned stars for three domains: (1) selection (maximum of four stars), (2) comparability (maximum of two stars), and (3) outcome (maximum of three stars). The selection domain includes "Representativeness of the exposed cohort", "Selection of the non-exposed cohort", "Ascertainment of exposure", and "Demonstration that outcome of interest was not present at start of study" to evaluate the accuracy of the experimental group definition, the representativeness of the patient group, and the appropriateness of the control group. The comparability domain includes "Comparability of cohorts on the basis of the design or analysis controlled for confounders". The outcome domain includes "Assessment of outcome", "Was follow-up long enough for outcomes to occur", and "Adequacy of follow-up of cohorts", to evaluate the outcome evaluation method, evaluation timing, and accuracy. Then, the overall score was obtained by adding up the number of stars acquired across the three domains.

Two reviewers independently assessed the included six studies. Any unresolved disagreements between reviewers were resolved by a discussion with the third author.

2.6. Statistical Analysis

This meta-analysis investigated the outcomes of patients with hip fractures during the COVID-19 pandemic compared to before the pandemic. We calculated the pooled odds ratio (OR) with a 95% confidence interval (CI) using a random-effects model for mortality, presented as a forest plot. To minimize the influence of other variables as much as possible, the unadjusted OR value was used. When raw data were presented in the paper, the unadjusted odds ratio was calculated using the presented values. We estimated the inter-study inconsistency using the I^2 test of the Higgins statistic to assess heterogeneity. Statistical heterogeneity was considered low if the I^2 value was less than 25%, moderate if it was between 25 and 50%, high if it was between 50 and 75%, and very high if it was more than 75%. After obtaining the OR of outcome, the pooled effect size was estimated using the inverse variance weighted method.

We conducted planned subgroup analyses on extracted subgroup variables for the sample size, study facility, and study period. We performed a meta-analysis using statistical analysis software R (version 4.0.0, The R Foundation for Statistical Computing, Vienna, Austria) and packages "meta" (version 4.11-0) and "metaphor" (version 2.1-0). A *p*-value <0.05 was considered statistically significant. We assessed for publication bias using a funnel plot.

3. Results

In total, we identified 820 studies, with 611 studies remaining after we removed duplicates. We excluded 40 studies for irrelevance after assessing their titles and abstracts and retrieved the full texts of the 95 remaining relevant studies. We then excluded studies that had an irrelevant population (n = 39), irrelevant control (n = 3), irrelevant outcome (n = 11), or duplicated data (n = 2). Finally, we conducted a meta-analysis and systematic review, including 40 eligible studies with 17,753 patients with hip fractures, among which were 2280 patients with COVID-19 (12.8%) [11,20–58]. Except for Vialonga et al. (2020), all studies had a research period in 2020 [54]. Hall et al. (2022) reported the highest number of COVID-19 infections with 651 [36], followed by Rashid et al. (2022) with 517 infections [50]. Among the studies that reported the frequency of surgery, Barker et al. (2021) had the lowest rate of surgical treatment, with only 60% performed [21]. In all reported studies, the frequency of female patients was higher than that of male patients. Notably, in Jiménez-Telleria et al. (2020), the frequency of male patients was as low as 21% [37]. Table 1 shows the baseline characteristics of included studies, and Figure 1 presents the study selection flowchart.

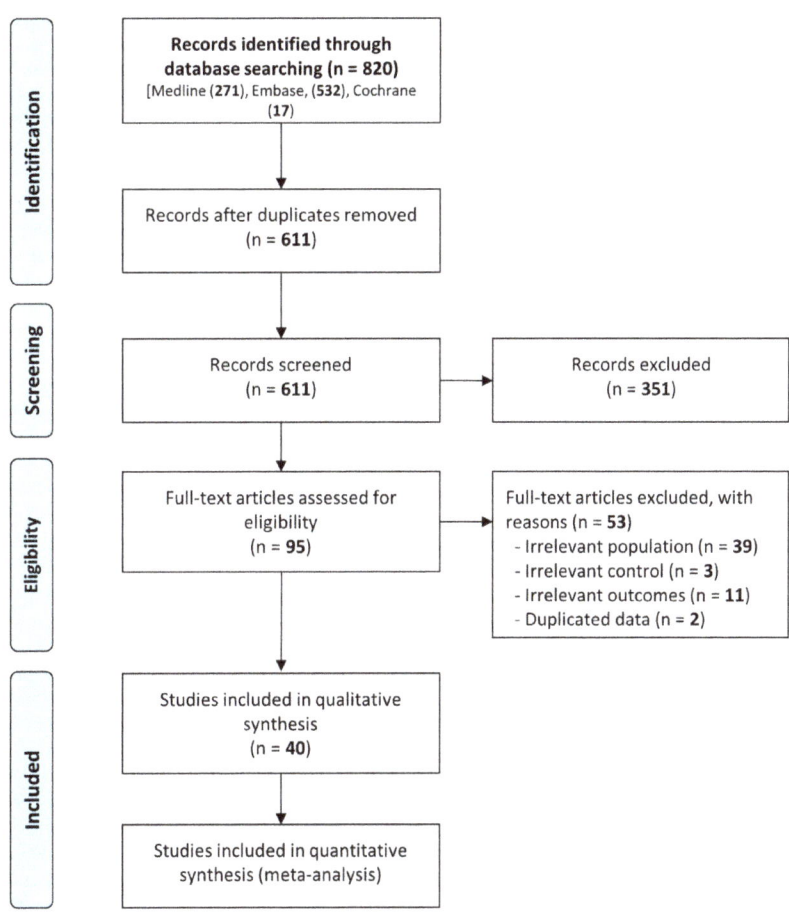

Figure 1. Flow diagram for the identification of relevant studies.

Table 1. Baseline characteristics of the included studies.

Study	Region	Period	Population		Age		Sex, Male,%		Rate of Operation		Length of Stay	
			COVID-19 +	COVID-19 −	+	−	+	−	+	−	+	−
Ali 2022 [20]	UK	March–June 2020	18	160	86	83	39	28	89	98	-	-
Arafa 2020 [11]	UK	1 March–31 May 2020	19	78	86 ± 8	83 ± 8	47	27	89	99	6 ± 1	5 ± 2
Barker 2021 [21]	UK	24 March–22 April 2020	5	61	-	-	-	-	60	100	-	-
Bayrak 2021 [22]	Turkey	April–November 2020	24	63	80 ± 15	79 ± 12	38	35	100	100	11 (9–16)	9 (7–11)
Beaven 2021 [23]	UK	28 March–25 May 2020	40	152	-	-	-	-	-	-	-	-
Biarnes-Sune 2021 [24]	Spain	11 March–24 April 2020	18	45	87 ± 7	85 ± 7	33	29	83	98	18 ± 9	11 ± 5

Table 1. Cont.

Study	Region	Period	Population		Age		Sex, Male,%		Rate of Operation		Length of Stay	
			COVID-19 +	COVID-19 −	+	-	+	-	+	-	+	-
Chan 2022 [25]	UK	1 March–30 April 2020	87	659	86	83	38	28	-	-	-	-
Chui 2020 [26]	UK	31 March–29 April 2020	6	41	-	-	-	-	100	100	-	-
Clement 2020 [27]	UK	1 March–19 April 2020	68	1501	-	-	-	-	91	100	-	-
Clough 2020 [28]	UK	23 March–15 June 2020	7	77	85 ± 8	78 ± 11	57	36	100	100	17 ± 11	14 ± 6
Cuthbert 2021 [29]	UK	1 February–21 May 2020	51	146	79 ± 11	77 ± 13	51	37	98	99	23 (19–31)	9 (7–13)
Dallari 2021 [30]	Italy	8 March–4 May 2020	53	424	83 ± 1	81 ± 1	9	22	100	100	15 ± 2	11
De 2021 [31]	UK	1 March–15 May 2020	9	20	81	83	38	27	94	99	-	-
Egol 2020 [32]	US	1 February–15 April 2020	31	107	82 ± 10	83 ± 10	52	32	85	100	10 ± 5	5 ± 3
Fadulelmola 2021 [33]	UK	March–April 2020	20	55	83	84	35	27	95	96	-	-
Fell 2021 [34]	UK	23 March–12 May 2020	11	44	90 ± 8	86 ± 8	55	27	-	-	7 ± 7	5 ± 6
Hall 2020 [35]	UK	1 March–15 April 2020	27	290	84 ± 11	80 ± 11	52	32	93	96	-	-
Hall 2022 [36]	14 nations	1 March–31 May 2020	651	6439	84 ± 9	82 ± 11	37	29	60	62	17 ± 13	10 ± 8
Jiménez-Telleria 2020 [37]	Spain	9 March–15 April 2020	10	67	85 ± 7	85 ± 8	10	21	90	97	11 (7–11)	6 (5–8)
Karayiannis 2020 [38]	UK	18 March–27 April 2020	27	176	-	-	-	-	100	100	-	-
Kayani 2020 [39]	UK	1 February–20 April 2020	82	340	72 ± 10	73 ± 7	38	40	100	100	14 ± 5	7 ± 3
LeBrun 2020 [40]	US	20 March–25 April 2020	9	50	87 ± 8	85 ± 8	33	24	78	100	8 (4–13)	6 (3–10)
Levitt 2022 [41]	US	15 March–31 December 2020	185	3118	83 ± 8	82 ± 8	40	32	100	100	25 ± 6	25 ± 5
Lim 2021 [42]	UK	1 March–15 May 2020	7	89	88 ± 4	85 ± 9	14	28	100	95	30 ± 17	12 ± 7
Macey 2020 [43]	UK	20 March–25 April 2020	10	66	-	-	-	-	-	-	-	-
Malik-Tabassum 2021 [44]	UK	23 March–11 May 2020	28	214	87 ± 8	83 ± 8	32	30	96	99	16 ± 10	12 ± 8
Mamrelis 2020 [45]	UK	1 March–30 April 2020	11	26	84 ± 10	78 ± 10	38	30	73	89	-	-
Maniscalco 2020 [46]	Italy	22 February–18 April 2020	32	89	-	-	-	-	-	-	-	-
Munoz Vives 2020 [47]	Spain	14 March–4 April 2020	23	39	-	-	-	-	-	-	-	-
Narang 2021 [48]	UK	1 March–30 April 2020	86	596	86	83	38	29	100	100	-	-
Oputa 2021 [49]	UK	5 March–5 April 2020	46	46	84 ± 7	82 ± 9	52	26	85	96	-	-
Rashid 2022 [50]	UK	23 March–31 December 2020	517	620	84	81 ± 10	35	31	99	97	24	13 ± 18
Segarra 2020 [51]	Spain	1 February–15 April 2020	2	66	88	82	50	32	100	944	7 ± 3	-
Sobti 2020 [52]	UK	1 March–31 May 2020	6	88	83	-	-	-	-	-	-	-
Thakrar 2020 [53]	UK	15 March–15 April 2020	12	6	-	-	-	-	-	-	-	-

Table 1. *Cont.*

Study	Region	Period	Population COVID-19 +	Population COVID-19 −	Age +	Age −	Sex, Male,% +	Sex, Male,% −	Rate of Operation +	Rate of Operation −	Length of Stay +	Length of Stay −
Vialonga 2020 [54]	US	March 2020–March 2021	15	134	74 ± 21	78 ± 16	27	27	-	-	10.1 ± 6.2	7 ± 4
Walters 2022 [55]	UK	17 February–17 May 2020	10	36	-	-	-	-	-	-	-	-
Wignall 2021 [56]	UK	1 March–30 May 2020	34	242	85 ± 8	81 ± 12	41	37	-	-	18 ± 9	15 ± 11
Wright 2021 [57]	UK	11 March–30 April 2020	10	58	81 ± 11	-	-	-	90	98.3	17 ± 6	10 ± 9
Zamora 2021 [58]	Chile	15 March–30 August 2020	24	138	81 (75–88)	81 (77–89)	17	14	87	100	12.5 (7–23)	6.5 (4–11)

3.1. Quality Assessment

We used the Newcastle–Ottawa Scale to evaluate article quality. All studies had four points in the selection domain and one point in outcome assessment, and 15 studies had an additional two points due to adjusting the confounding factors (Supplementary Table S2).

3.2. Overall and Regional Mortality of Patients with Hip Fractures during the COVID-19 Pandemic

The pooled 30-day mortality was 12.6% (95% CI 10.6–14.9%, $I^2 = 90\%$) during the COVID-19 pandemic for the 40 included studies involving 17,753 hip fractures (Figure 2). In the United Kingdom, the 30-day mortality of hip fractures during the pandemic was 14.3%; in Spain, it was 14.9%; in Italy, it was 9.6%; and in the United States (US), it was 6.2%.

3.3. Comparison of Pooled Mortality for Hip Fractures between Those with and without COVID-19

We conducted a meta-analysis of patients with hip fractures between those with and without COVID-19 from the 40 included studies. Those with COVID-19 had significantly increased mortality compared to patients who did not have COVID-19 (OR, 7.10; 95% CI, 5.51–9.15; $I^2 = 57\%$; Figure 3).

3.4. Subgroup Analysis

We performed a subgroup analysis according to sample size (100 or more, or fewer than 100), study facility (single center or multi-center), and study period (the beginning of the pandemic or other periods). In all of the subgroup analyses, the 30-day mortality rates were significantly increased in those with hip fractures who had COVID-19 compared to those without COVID-19. Studies with fewer than 100 patients and in a single center were low-heterogeneity (12% and 19%) (Table 2).

3.5. Publication Bias

The funnel plot demonstrated symmetry, and we did not find publication bias in the included studies (Supplementary Figure S1).

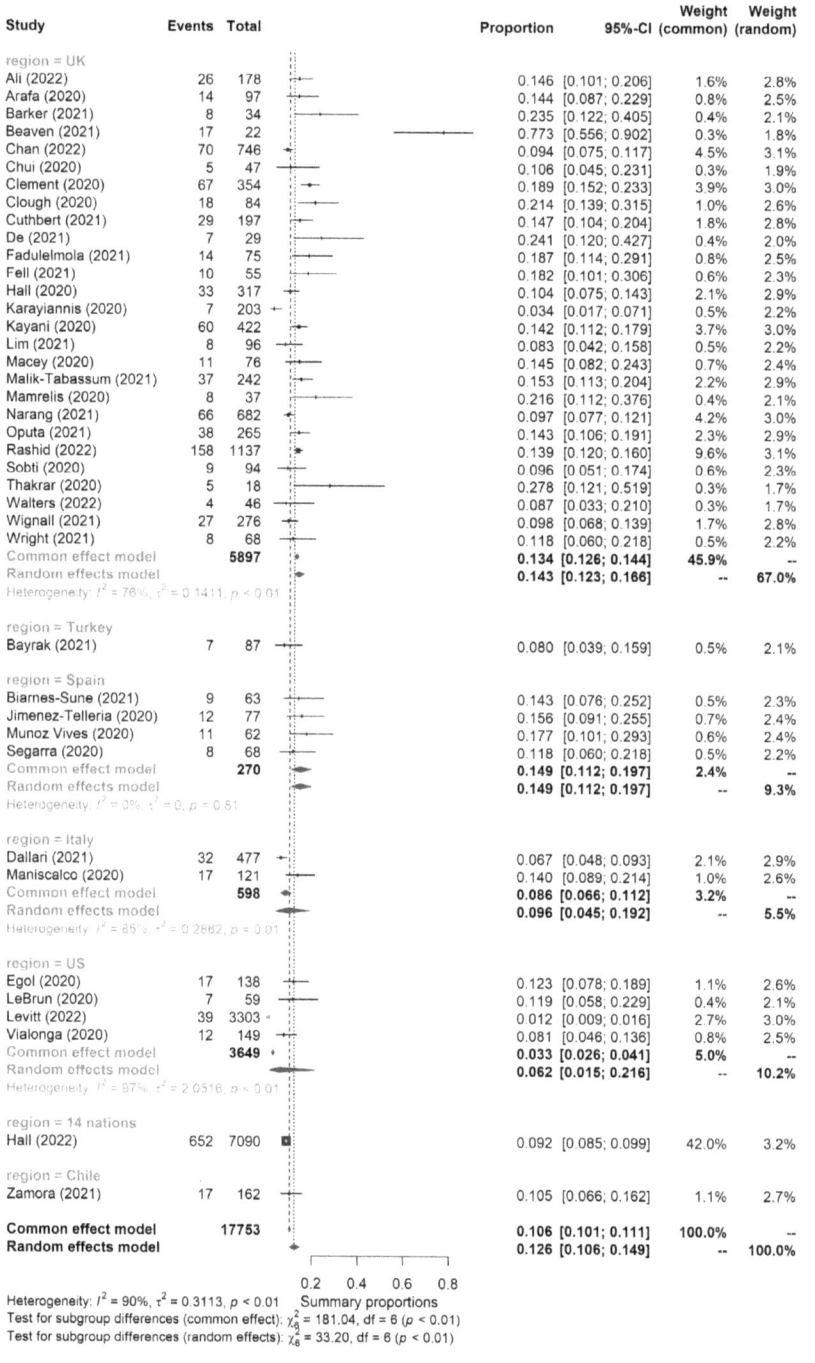

Figure 2. Forest plot for 30-day mortality of patients with hip fractures during the COVID-19 pandemic according to the study region [11,20–58].

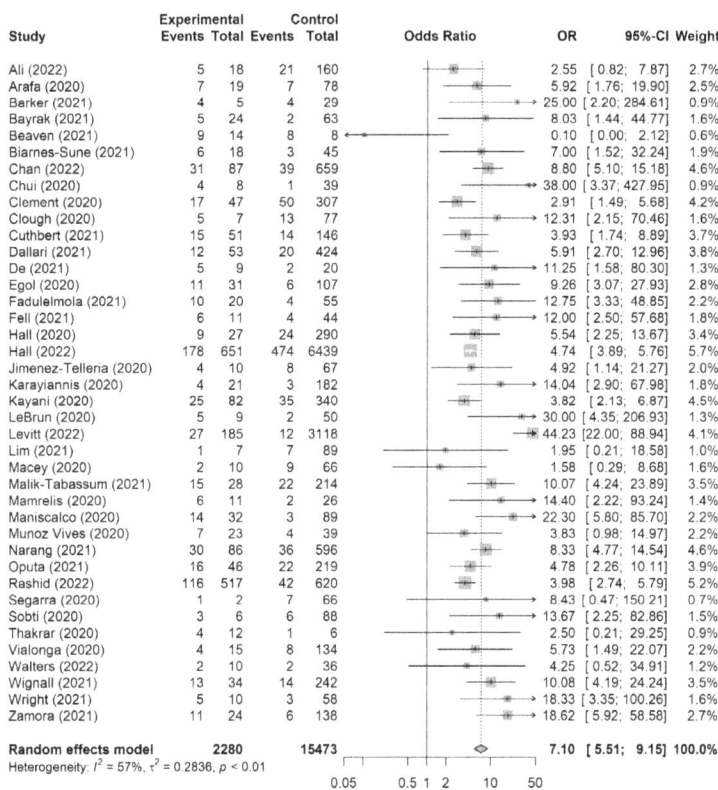

Figure 3. Forest plot for meta-analysis of patients with hip fractures with and without COVID-19 [11,20–58].

Table 2. Subgroup analysis for the 30-day mortality of hip fractures in patients with and without COVID-19.

Characteristics	The 30-Day Mortality			
	N	OR (95% CI)	p-Value for Heterogeneity	I^2, %
All	40	7.10 (5.51–9.15)	<0.01	57
Population				
≥100	19	6.99 (5.03–9.71)	<0.01	73
<100	21	7.50 (5.09–11.03)	0.30	12
Facility				
Single center	18	6.16 (4.08–9.30)	0.22	19
Multi-center	22	7.54 (5.50–10.34)	<0.01	70
Period				
Beginning of the pandemic	33	6.34 (5.13–7.84)	0.04	32
Other periods	7	9.04 (3.96–20.68)	<0.01	86
Region				
United Kingdom	27	5.92 (4.63–7.58)	0.02	38
Spain	4	5.18 (2.32–11.56)	0.93	0
Italy	2	10.21 (2.84–36.73)	0.10	64
United States	4	16.87 (6.03–47.07)	0.02	70

4. Discussion

As the COVID-19 pandemic unfolds, it is crucial to monitor the impact on healthcare systems and patient outcomes. The present study shows that the 30-day mortality rate for patients with hip fractures is significantly higher in those with COVID-19 infection. The 30-day mortality rate for patients with hip fractures during the COVID-19 pandemic was 12.6% in a meta-analysis, which is similar to previous studies (Clement et al., 2020; 13%) [15]. Factors such as hospital arrival delays, unequal allocation of medical resources, and limited surgical interventions to minimize the spread of infection must be accounted for to effectively manage patients with hip fractures during the pandemic [59,60]. Effective infection control measures, prioritizing high-risk patients, and proper communication and coordination between healthcare providers help ensure optimal outcomes for these patients during the pandemic [59,61,62].

The COVID-19 pandemic has had a profound impact on the mortality rates and healthcare systems of many countries. Previous meta-analyses mainly analyzed data from the UK, but this study aimed to evaluate mortalities by country [15,16]. The mortality rate in the UK was 14.3%, with Spain and Italy at 14.9% and 9.6%, respectively. In the US, four studies showed a mortality rate of 6.2%. The mortality rates of those infected with COVID-19 in the UK, Spain, Italy, and the US were 30.5%, 34.0%, 30.6%, and 20.8%, respectively, and the ORs were all significantly high (5.92, 5.18, 10.21, and 16.87, respectively). It is clear that COVID-19 infection increases the 30-day mortality of hip fractures.

In Europe, shortages of hospital beds, medical supplies, and staff early in the COVID-19 pandemic affected the mortality rate of patients with hip fractures. The 30-day mortality rates of patients with hip fractures were 1.4–10% in the 15 included studies of Giannoulis et al. (2016) [63], demonstrating that this 30-day mortality increased considerably during the pandemic. The UK's initial strategy focused on herd immunity, but lockdowns were implemented as the situation worsened [64]. In Italy, strict lockdowns and other measures to halt the spread of the virus were necessary due to medical supply shortages and high numbers of patients [65,66]. In the US, the first COVID-19 wave was intense, leading to a widely criticized shortage of personal protective equipment and an overwhelmed healthcare system [67]. Conversely, South Korea, China, and Japan had lower mortality rates due to prompt pandemic management and a more robust healthcare system and infrastructure [68]. Pandemic responses and management varied widely across countries, depending on their healthcare system, economic stability, and government policies [64,67,68]. The most valuable lesson from Asia is the ability to prevent pandemics through improved hygiene and isolation of infectious individuals, as opposed to relying on severe economic shutdowns [69]. Several Asian countries have shown superlative results in suppressing the virus and keeping death rates per million incredibly low [69]. They learned from their experiences of the coronavirus that causes Severe Acute Respiratory Syndrome and favored rapid lockdowns or intensive mass testing and contact tracing without the need for a full-scale lockdown [70]. These different circumstances were reflected by the increase in the 30-day mortality rate of hip fractures.

However, the 30-day mortality of hip fractures in patients who did not have COVID-19 during the pandemic has not changed significantly. In this study, the mortality rate of patients without COVID-19 during the pandemic was similar to that of previous hip fracture deaths (Total: 6.13%, UK: 8.4%, Spain: 10.1%, Italy: 4.5%, and the US: 0.8%). After the first COVID-19 wave, the decrease in activity and the total number of patients indicated the possibility of increasing the emergency capacity for non-COVID-19 patients and providing efficient treatment. In addition, previous studies indicated that COVID-19 was a new mortality risk factor [27,35], and the high risk of COVID-19 infection during the pandemic increased the infection risk in patients with hip fractures. The direct effect of hip fracture on 30-day mortality is likely low.

This analysis revealed a prolonged research period, including the early stages of the pandemic, and included many patients. Several studies collected data from multiple institutions and countries through a registry, and Levitt et al. (2022) studied hip fracture mortality using nationwide data in the United States [41]. However, most of the included studies only encompassed data from the early stages of the pandemic. The pandemic is ongoing, so this analysis may not reflect the current medical system or account for the existing mortality rate of hip fractures due to COVID-19. Rashid et al. (2022) investigated the 30-day mortality of patients with hip fractures diagnosed with COVID-19 in the first and second waves and statistically confirmed a decrease in mortality in the second wave [50]. Although seven studies were conducted after the first wave, they included patients from the first wave. Future studies should examine the changes in mortality based on the pandemic period.

There are several limitations to this analysis. First, the study institutions' medical resources were inadequately assessed. The medical resources available at each institution during the pandemic could not be determined, which could impact their response to patients with hip fractures. There was no information on whether patient accommodations were restricted or if examinations and treatments were limited. Second, it is difficult to generalize outcomes due to the limited study regions. This study is limited to Europe, with most data coming from the UK. Few studies were conducted in Asia, making it difficult to generalize these results. Third, most studies focused on the early pandemic stages, and only seven studies were conducted in the later pandemic stages. One case was classified by period, but the entire pandemic period should be analyzed at specific time points to account for the development of vaccines, therapeutic agents, and viral variants [63]. Finally, there were insufficient data on fracture types and comorbidities from the included studies. In some studies, the fracture type or underlying condition was reported, but lack of information prevented the collection of all relevant evidence. Future research requires a review based on a comprehensive investigation of this issue.

5. Conclusions

Patients with hip fractures who have COVID-19 have a significantly higher 30-day mortality rate than those without COVID-19. COVID-19 infection may have contributed to the increase in 30-day mortality for patients with hip fractures. The overall 30-day mortality rate for patients with hip fractures during the COVID-19 pandemic was 12.6%. Mortality rates varied by country, with Europe, including the UK and Spain, having the highest mortality rates.

Factors such as hospital arrival delays, unequal allocation of medical resources, and limited surgical interventions to minimize the spread of infection must be considered to effectively manage patients with hip fractures during the pandemic. Implementing effective infection control measures, prioritizing high-risk patients, and ensuring proper communication and coordination between healthcare providers can help achieve optimal outcomes for these patients. Future studies should systematically analyze these factors and track changes in mortality rates over time while investigating different pandemic periods.

Supplementary Materials: The following supporting information can be downloaded at: https://www.mdpi.com/article/10.3390/jpm13040669/s1, Figure S1: Funnel plot for assessment of publication bias; Table S1: Search strategy (Search on 27 November 2022). Table S2: Quality assessments of individual studies.

Author Contributions: Conceptualization, S.H. and C.A.; methodology, M.W. and C.A.; investigation, S.H. and C.A.; data curation, S.H. and C.A.; writing—original draft preparation, S.H. and C.A.; writing—review and editing, all authors; visualization, M.W. and C.A.; supervision, C.A. All authors have read and agreed to the published version of the manuscript.

Funding: This research received no external funding.

Institutional Review Board Statement: Not applicable.

Informed Consent Statement: Not applicable.

Data Availability Statement: The datasets generated during the current study are available from the corresponding author on reasonable request.

Conflicts of Interest: The authors declare no conflict of interest.

References

1. Choi, A.; Kim, H.Y.; Cho, A.; Noh, J.; Park, I.; Chung, H.S. Efficacy of a four-tier infection response system in the emergency department during the coronavirus disease-2019 outbreak. *PLoS ONE* **2021**, *16*, e0256116. [CrossRef] [PubMed]
2. Blumenthal, D.; Fowler, E.J.; Abrams, M.; Collins, S.R. Covid-19—Implications for the Health Care System. *N. Engl. J. Med.* **2020**, *383*, 1483–1488. [CrossRef] [PubMed]
3. Kim, J.H.; Ahn, C.; Namgung, M. Comparative Evaluation of the Prognosis of Septic Shock Patients from Before to After the Onset of the COVID-19 Pandemic: A Retrospective Single-Center Clinical Analysis. *J. Pers. Med.* **2022**, *12*, 103. [CrossRef] [PubMed]
4. Ahn, J.Y.; Ryoo, H.W.; Cho, J.W.; Kim, J.H.; Lee, S.H.; Jang, T.C. Impact of the COVID-19 outbreak on adult out-of-hospital cardiac arrest outcomes in Daegu, South Korea: An observational study. *Clin. Exp. Emerg. Med.* **2021**, *8*, 137–144. [CrossRef]
5. Lange, S.J.; Ritchey, M.D.; Goodman, A.B.; Dias, T.; Twentyman, E.; Fuld, J.; Schieve, L.A.; Imperatore, G.; Benoit, S.R.; Kite-Powell, A.; et al. Potential indirect effects of the COVID-19 pandemic on use of emergency departments for acute life-threatening conditions—United States, January–May 2020. *Am. J. Transplant.* **2020**, *20*, 2612–2617. [CrossRef]
6. Furnica, C.; Chistol, R.O.; Chiran, D.A.; Stan, C.I.; Sargu, G.D.; Girlescu, N.; Tinica, G. The Impact of the Early COVID-19 Pandemic on ST-Segment Elevation Myocardial Infarction Presentation and Outcomes-A Systematic Review and Meta-Analysis. *Diagnostics* **2022**, *12*, 588. [CrossRef]
7. Ishaque, N.; Butt, A.J.; Kamtchum-Tatuene, J.; Nomani, A.Z.; Razzaq, S.; Fatima, N.; Vekhande, C.; Nair, R.; Akhtar, N.; Khan, K.; et al. Trends in Stroke Presentations before and during the COVID-19 Pandemic: A Meta-Analysis. *J. Stroke* **2022**, *24*, 65–78. [CrossRef]
8. Lim, Z.J.; Ponnapa Reddy, M.; Afroz, A.; Billah, B.; Shekar, K.; Subramaniam, A. Incidence and outcome of out-of-hospital cardiac arrests in the COVID-19 era: A systematic review and meta-analysis. *Resuscitation* **2020**, *157*, 248–258. [CrossRef]
9. Kim, J.H.; Ahn, C.; Namgung, M. Epidemiology and Outcome of Out-of-Hospital Cardiac Arrests during the COVID-19 Pandemic in South Korea: A Systematic Review and Meta-Analyses. *Yonsei Med. J.* **2022**, *63*, 1121–1129. [CrossRef]
10. Köhler, F.; Müller, S.; Hendricks, A.; Kastner, C.; Reese, L.; Boerner, K.; Flemming, S.; Lock, J.F.; Germer, C.T.; Wiegering, A. Changes in appendicitis treatment during the COVID-19 pandemic—A systematic review and meta-analysis. *Int. J. Surg.* **2021**, *95*, 106148. [CrossRef]
11. Arafa, M.; Nesar, S.; Abu-Jabeh, H.; Jayme, M.O.R.; Kalairajah, Y. COVID-19 pandemic and hip fractures: Impact and lessons learned. *Bone Jt. Open* **2020**, *1*, 530–540. [CrossRef]
12. National_Office_of_Clinical_Audit. Irish Hip Fracture Database National Report 2019. Available online: https://www.noca.ie/documents/ihfd-national-report-2019 (accessed on 12 February 2023).
13. Haskel, J.D.; Lin, C.C.; Kaplan, D.J.; Dankert, J.F.; Merkow, D.; Crespo, A.; Behery, O.; Ganta, A.; Konda, S.R. Hip Fracture Volume Does Not Change at a New York City Level 1 Trauma Center During a Period of Social Distancing. *Geriatr. Orthop. Surg. Rehabil.* **2020**, *11*, 2151459320972674. [CrossRef] [PubMed]
14. Ojeda-Thies, C.; Cuarental-García, J.; García-Gómez, E.; Salazar-Zamorano, C.H.; Alberti-Maroño, J.; Ramos-Pascua, L.R. Hip fracture care and mortality among patients treated in dedicated COVID-19 and non-COVID-19 circuits. *Eur. Geriatr. Med.* **2021**, *12*, 749–757. [CrossRef] [PubMed]
15. Clement, N.D.; Ng, N.; Simpson, C.J.; Patton, R.F.L.; Hall, A.J.; Simpson, A.; Duckworth, A.D. The prevalence, mortality, and associated risk factors for developing COVID-19 in hip fracture patients: A systematic review and meta-analysis. *Bone Jt. Res.* **2020**, *9*, 873–883. [CrossRef] [PubMed]
16. Patralekh, M.K.; Jain, V.K.; Iyengar, K.P.; Upadhyaya, G.K.; Vaishya, R. Mortality escalates in patients of proximal femoral fractures with COVID-19: A systematic review and meta-analysis of 35 studies on 4255 patients. *J. Clin. Orthop. Trauma* **2021**, *18*, 80–93. [CrossRef] [PubMed]
17. Liberati, A.; Altman, D.G.; Tetzlaff, J.; Mulrow, C.; Gøtzsche, P.C.; Ioannidis, J.P.; Clarke, M.; Devereaux, P.J.; Kleijnen, J.; Moher, D. The PRISMA statement for reporting systematic reviews and meta-analyses of studies that evaluate healthcare interventions: Explanation and elaboration. *BMJ* **2009**, *339*, b2700. [CrossRef]
18. Stroup, D.F.; Berlin, J.A.; Morton, S.C.; Olkin, I.; Williamson, G.D.; Rennie, D.; Moher, D.; Becker, B.J.; Sipe, T.A.; Thacker, S.B. Meta-analysis of observational studies in epidemiology: A proposal for reporting. Meta-analysis Of Observational Studies in Epidemiology (MOOSE) group. *JAMA* **2000**, *283*, 2008–2012. [CrossRef]
19. Wells, G.A.; Shea, B.; O'Connell, D.; Peterson, J.; Welch, V.; Losos, M.; Tugwell, P. The Newcastle-Ottawa Scale (NOS) for Assessing the Quality of Nonrandomised Studies in Meta-Analyses. Available online: https://www.ohri.ca/programs/clinical_epidemiology/oxford.asp (accessed on 12 February 2023).
20. Ali, M.; Fadulelmola, A.; Urwin, M.; Nita, C. Achieving the hip fracture Best Practise Tariff during the COVID-19 pandemic. *J. Frailty Sarcopenia Falls* **2022**, *7*, 13–17. [CrossRef]
21. Barker, T.; Thompson, J.; Corbett, J.; Johal, S.; McNamara, I. Increased 30-day mortality rate in patients admitted with hip fractures during the COVID-19 pandemic in the UK. *Eur. J. Trauma Emerg. Surg.* **2021**, *47*, 1327–1334. [CrossRef]
22. Bayrak, A.; Duramaz, A.; Çakmak, B.B.; Kural, C.; Basaran, S.H.; Erçin, E.; Kural, A.; Ursavaş, H.T. The effect of COVID-19 positivity on inflammatory parameters and thirty-day mortality rates in patients over sixty-five years of age with surgically treated intertrochanteric fractures. *Int. Orthop.* **2021**, *45*, 3025–3031. [CrossRef]

23. Beaven, A.; Piper, D.; Plant, C.; Sharma, A.; Agrawal, Y.; Cooper, G. Thirty-Day Mortality for Proximal Femoral Fractures Treated at a U.K. Elective Center with a Site-Streaming Policy During the COVID-19 Pandemic. *JB JS Open Access* **2021**, *6*. [CrossRef] [PubMed]
24. Biarnés-Suñé, A.; Solà-Enríquez, B.; González Posada, M.; Teixidor-Serra, J.; García-Sánchez, Y.; Manrique Muñóz, S. Impact of the COVID-19 pandemic on the mortality of the elderly patient with a hip fracture. *Rev. Esp. Anestesiol. Reanim. (Engl. Ed.)* **2021**, *68*, 65–72. [CrossRef] [PubMed]
25. Chan, G.; Narang, A.; Aframian, A.; Ali, Z.; Bridgeman, J.; Carr, A.; Chapman, L.; Goodier, H.; Morgan, C.; Park, C.; et al. Medium-term mortality after hip fractures and COVID-19: A prospective multi-centre UK study. *Chin. J. Traumatol.* **2022**, *25*, 161–165. [CrossRef] [PubMed]
26. Chui, K.; Thakrar, A.; Shankar, S. Evaluating the efficacy of a two-site ('COVID-19' and 'COVID-19-free') trauma and orthopaedic service for the management of hip fractures during the COVID-19 pandemic in the UK. *Bone Jt. Open* **2020**, *1*, 190–197. [CrossRef] [PubMed]
27. Clement, N.D.; Hall, A.J.; Makaram, N.S.; Robinson, P.G.; Patton, R.F.L.; Moran, M.; Macpherson, G.J.; Duckworth, A.D.; Jenkins, P.J. IMPACT-Restart: The influence of COVID-19 on postoperative mortality and risk factors associated with SARS-CoV-2 infection after orthopaedic and trauma surgery. *Bone Jt. J.* **2020**, *102-b*, 1774–1781. [CrossRef]
28. Clough, T.M.; Shah, N.; Divecha, H.; Talwalkar, S. COVID-19 consent and return to elective orthopaedic surgery: Allowing a true patient choice? *Bone Jt. Open* **2020**, *1*, 556–561. [CrossRef]
29. Cuthbert, R.; Ferguson, D.; Kayani, B.; Haque, S.; Ali, A.; Parkar, A.; Bates, P.; Vemulapalli, K. Evidence-based approach to providing informed consent for hip fracture surgery during the COVID-19 era. *World J. Orthop.* **2021**, *12*, 386–394. [CrossRef]
30. Dallari, D.; Zagra, L.; Cimatti, P.; Guindani, N.; D'Apolito, R.; Bove, F.; Casiraghi, A.; Catani, F.; D'Angelo, F.; Franceschini, M.; et al. Early mortality in hip fracture patients admitted during the first wave of the COVID-19 pandemic in Northern Italy: A multicentre study. *J. Orthop. Traumatol.* **2021**, *22*, 15. [CrossRef]
31. De, C.; Harbham, P.K.; Postoyalko, C.; Bhavanasi, B.; Paringe, V.; Theivendran, K. Mortality Following Hip Fracture Surgery During COVID-19 Pandemic Compared to Pre-COVID-19 Period: A Case Matched Cohort Series. *Malays. Orthop. J.* **2021**, *15*, 107–114. [CrossRef]
32. Egol, K.A.; Konda, S.R.; Bird, M.L.; Dedhia, N.; Landes, E.K.; Ranson, R.A.; Solasz, S.J.; Aggarwal, V.K.; Bosco, J.A., 3rd; Furgiuele, D.L.; et al. Increased Mortality and Major Complications in Hip Fracture Care During the COVID-19 Pandemic: A New York City Perspective. *J. Orthop. Trauma* **2020**, *34*, 395–402. [CrossRef]
33. Fadulelmola, A.; Gregory, R.; Gordon, G.; Smith, F.; Jennings, A. The impact of COVID-19 infection on hip fractures 30-day mortality. *Trauma* **2021**, *23*, 295–300. [CrossRef]
34. Fell, A.; Malik-Tabassum, K.; Rickman, S.; Arealis, G. Thirty-day mortality and reliability of Nottingham Hip Fracture Score in patients with COVID-19 infection. *J. Orthop.* **2021**, *26*, 111–114. [CrossRef]
35. Hall, A.J.; Clement, N.D.; Farrow, L.; MacLullich, A.M.J.; Dall, G.F.; Scott, C.E.H.; Jenkins, P.J.; White, T.O.; Duckworth, A.D. IMPACT-Scot report on COVID-19 and hip fractures. *Bone Jt. J.* **2020**, *102-b*, 1219–1228. [CrossRef]
36. Hall, A.J.; Clement, N.D.; Ojeda-Thies, C.; MacLullich, A.M.; Toro, G.; Johansen, A.; White, T.O.; Duckworth, A.D. IMPACT-Global Hip Fracture Audit: Nosocomial infection, risk prediction and prognostication, minimum reporting standards and global collaborative audit: Lessons from an international multicentre study of 7090 patients conducted in 14 nations during the COVID-19 pandemic. *Surgeon* **2022**, *20*, e429–e446. [CrossRef] [PubMed]
37. Jiménez-Tellería, I.; Urra, I.; Fernández-Gutiérrez, L.; Aragon, E.; Aguirre, U.; Foruria, X.; Moreta, J. Thirty-day mortality in patients with a proximal femur fracture during the COVID-19 pandemic in Biscay (Basque Country). *Rev. Esp. Cir. Ortop. Traumatol.* **2022**, *66*, 251–259. [CrossRef] [PubMed]
38. Karayiannis, P.N.; Roberts, V.; Cassidy, R.; Mayne, A.I.W.; McAuley, D.; Milligan, D.J.; Diamond, O. 30-day mortality following trauma and orthopaedic surgery during the peak of the COVID-19 pandemic: A multicentre regional analysis of 484 patients. *Bone Jt. Open* **2020**, *1*, 392–397. [CrossRef] [PubMed]
39. Kayani, B.; Onochie, E.; Patil, V.; Begum, F.; Cuthbert, R.; Ferguson, D.; Bhamra, J.S.; Sharma, A.; Bates, P.; Haddad, F.S. The effects of COVID-19 on perioperative morbidity and mortality in patients with hip fractures. *Bone Jt. J.* **2020**, *102-b*, 1136–1145. [CrossRef] [PubMed]
40. LeBrun, D.G.; Konnaris, M.A.; Ghahramani, G.C.; Premkumar, A.; DeFrancesco, C.J.; Gruskay, J.A.; Dvorzhinskiy, A.; Sandhu, M.S.; Goldwyn, E.M.; Mendias, C.L.; et al. Hip Fracture Outcomes During the COVID-19 Pandemic: Early Results From New York. *J. Orthop. Trauma* **2020**, *34*, 403–410. [CrossRef]
41. Levitt, E.B.; Patch, D.A.; Mabry, S.; Terrero, A.; Jaeger, B.; Haendel, M.A.; Chute, C.G.; Quade, J.H.; Ponce, B.; Theiss, S.; et al. Association Between COVID-19 and Mortality in Hip Fracture Surgery in the National COVID Cohort Collaborative (N3C): A Retrospective Cohort Study. *J. Am. Acad. Orthop. Surg. Glob. Res. Rev.* **2022**, *6*, e21.00282. [CrossRef]
42. Lim, J.A.; Thahir, A.; Amar Korde, V.; Krkovic, M. The Impact of COVID-19 on Neck of Femur Fracture Care: A Major Trauma Centre Experience, United Kingdom. *Arch. Bone Jt. Surg.* **2021**, *9*, 453–460. [CrossRef]
43. Macey, A.R.M.; Butler, J.; Martin, S.C.; Tan, T.Y.; Leach, W.J.; Jamal, B. 30-day outcomes in hip fracture patients during the COVID-19 pandemic compared to the preceding year. *Bone Jt. Open* **2020**, *1*, 415–419. [CrossRef] [PubMed]

44. Malik-Tabassum, K.; Robertson, A.; Tadros, B.J.; Chan, G.; Crooks, M.; Buckle, C.; Rogers, B.; Selmon, G.; Arealis, G. The effect of the COVID-19 lockdown on the epidemiology of hip fractures in the elderly: A multicentre cohort study. *Ann. R. Coll. Surg. Engl.* **2021**, *103*, 337–344. [CrossRef] [PubMed]
45. Mamarelis, G.; Oduoza, U.; Chekuri, R.; Estfan, R.; Greer, T. Mortality in Patients with Proximal Femoral Fracture During the COVID-19 Pandemic: A U.K. Hospital's Experience. *JB JS Open Access* **2020**, *5*, e20.00086. [CrossRef] [PubMed]
46. Maniscalco, P.; Poggiali, E.; Quattrini, F.; Ciatti, C.; Magnacavallo, A.; Vercelli, A.; Domenichini, M.; Vaienti, E.; Pogliacomi, F.; Ceccarelli, F. Proximal femur fractures in COVID-19 emergency: The experience of two Orthopedics and Traumatology Departments in the first eight weeks of the Italian epidemic. *Acta Biomed.* **2020**, *91*, 89–96. [CrossRef] [PubMed]
47. Muñoz Vives, J.M.; Jornet-Gibert, M.; Cámara-Cabrera, J.; Esteban, P.L.; Brunet, L.; Delgado-Flores, L.; Camacho-Carrasco, P.; Torner, P.; Marcano-Fernández, F. Mortality Rates of Patients with Proximal Femoral Fracture in a Worldwide Pandemic: Preliminary Results of the Spanish HIP-COVID Observational Study. *J. Bone Jt. Surg. Am.* **2020**, *102*, e69. [CrossRef] [PubMed]
48. Narang, A.; Chan, G.; Aframian, A.; Ali, Z.; Carr, A.; Goodier, H.; Morgan, C.; Park, C.; Sugand, K.; Walton, T.; et al. Thirty-day mortality following surgical management of hip fractures during the COVID-19 pandemic: Findings from a prospective multi-centre UK study. *Int. Orthop.* **2021**, *45*, 23–31. [CrossRef]
49. Oputa, T.J.; Dupley, L.; Bourne, J.T. One Hundred Twenty-Day Mortality Rates for Hip Fracture Patients with COVID-19 Infection. *Clin. Orthop. Surg.* **2021**, *13*, 135–143. [CrossRef]
50. Rashid, F.; Hawkes, D.; Mahmood, A.; Harrison, W.J. Hip fracture mortality in patients co-infected with coronavirus disease 2019: A comparison of the first two waves of the United Kingdom pandemic during the pre-vaccine era. *Int. Orthop.* **2022**, *46*, 171–178. [CrossRef]
51. Segarra, B.; Ballesteros Heras, N.; Viadel Ortiz, M.; Ribes-Iborra, J.; Martinez-Macias, O.; Cuesta-Peredo, D. Are Hospitals Safe? A Prospective Study on SARS-CoV-2 Prevalence and Outcome on Surgical Fracture Patients: A Closer Look at Hip Fracture Patients. *J. Orthop. Trauma* **2020**, *34*, e371–e376. [CrossRef]
52. Sobti, A.; Memon, K.; Bhaskar, R.R.P.; Unnithan, A.; Khaleel, A. Outcome of trauma and orthopaedic surgery at a UK District General Hospital during the Covid-19 pandemic. *J. Clin. Orthop. Trauma* **2020**, *11*, S442–S445. [CrossRef]
53. Thakrar, A.; Chui, K.; Kapoor, A.; Hambidge, J. Thirty-Day Mortality Rate of Patients With Hip Fractures During the COVID-19 Pandemic: A Single Centre Prospective Study in the United Kingdom. *J. Orthop. Trauma* **2020**, *34*, e325–e329. [CrossRef] [PubMed]
54. Vialonga, M.D.; Menken, L.G.; Tang, A.; Yurek, J.W.; Sun, L.; Feldman, J.J.; Liporace, F.A.; Yoon, R.S. Survivorship Analysis in Asymptomatic COVID-19+ Hip Fracture Patients: Is There an Increase in Mortality? *Hip Pelvis* **2022**, *34*, 25–34. [CrossRef] [PubMed]
55. Walters, S.; Raja, H.; Ahmad, R.; Tsitskaris, K. Short-Term Hip Fracture Outcomes during the COVID-19 Pandemic. *Surg. J. (N. Y.)* **2022**, *8*, e8–e13. [CrossRef] [PubMed]
56. Wignall, A.; Giannoudis, V.; De, C.; Jimenez, A.; Sturdee, S.; Nisar, S.; Pandit, H.; Gulati, A.; Palan, J. The impact of COVID-19 on the management and outcomes of patients with proximal femoral fractures: A multi-centre study of 580 patients. *J. Orthop. Surg. Res.* **2021**, *16*, 155. [CrossRef] [PubMed]
57. Wright, E.V.; Musbahi, O.; Singh, A.; Somashekar, N.; Huber, C.P.; Wiik, A.V. Increased perioperative mortality for femoral neck fractures in patients with coronavirus disease 2019 (COVID-19): Experience from the United Kingdom during the first wave of the pandemic. *Patient Saf. Surg.* **2021**, *15*, 8. [CrossRef]
58. Zamora, T.; Sandoval, F.; Demandes, H.; Serrano, J.; Gonzalez, J.; Lira, M.J.; Klaber, I.; Carmona, M.; Botello, E.; Schweitzer, D. Hip Fractures in the Elderly During the COVID-19 Pandemic: A Latin-American Perspective With a Minimum 90-Day Follow-Up. *Geriatr. Orthop. Surg. Rehabil.* **2021**, *12*, 21514593211024509. [CrossRef] [PubMed]
59. Chung, J.W.; Ha, Y.C.; Lee, M.K.; Kim, J.H.; Park, J.W.; Koo, K.H. Hip Fracture Management during the COVID-19 Pandemic in South Korea. *Clin. Orthop. Surg.* **2021**, *13*, 474–481. [CrossRef]
60. Jarvis, S.; Salottolo, K.; Madayag, R.; Pekarek, J.; Nwafo, N.; Wessel, A.; Duane, T.; Roberts, Z.; Lieser, M.; Corrigan, C.; et al. Delayed hospital admission for traumatic hip fractures during the COVID-19 pandemic. *J. Orthop. Surg. Res.* **2021**, *16*, 237. [CrossRef]
61. Qin, H.C.; He, Z.; Luo, Z.W.; Zhu, Y.L. Management of hip fracture in COVID-19 infected patients. *World J. Orthop.* **2022**, *13*, 544–554. [CrossRef]
62. Malik-Tabassum, K.; Crooks, M.; Robertson, A.; To, C.; Maling, L.; Selmon, G. Management of hip fractures during the COVID-19 pandemic at a high-volume hip fracture unit in the United Kingdom. *J. Orthop.* **2020**, *20*, 332–337. [CrossRef]
63. Ahn, C. Suggestions for the focus of OHCA meta-analysis in the COVID-19 era. *Resuscitation* **2022**, *174*, 20–21. [CrossRef] [PubMed]
64. Alanezi, F.; Aljahdali, A.; Alyousef, S.M.; Alrashed, H.; Mushcab, H.; AlThani, B.; Alghamedy, F.; Alotaibi, H.; Saadah, A.; Alanzi, T. A Comparative Study on the Strategies Adopted by the United Kingdom, India, China, Italy, and Saudi Arabia to Contain the Spread of the COVID-19 Pandemic. *J. Healthc. Leadersh.* **2020**, *12*, 117–131. [CrossRef] [PubMed]
65. Armocida, B.; Formenti, B.; Ussai, S.; Palestra, F.; Missoni, E. The Italian health system and the COVID-19 challenge. *Lancet Public Health* **2020**, *5*, e253. [CrossRef] [PubMed]
66. Ceylan, Z. Estimation of COVID-19 prevalence in Italy, Spain, and France. *Sci. Total. Environ.* **2020**, *729*, 138817. [CrossRef] [PubMed]

67. Unruh, L.; Allin, S.; Marchildon, G.; Burke, S.; Barry, S.; Siersbaek, R.; Thomas, S.; Rajan, S.; Koval, A.; Alexander, M.; et al. A comparison of 2020 health policy responses to the COVID-19 pandemic in Canada, Ireland, the United Kingdom and the United States of America. *Health Policy* **2022**, *126*, 427–437. [CrossRef] [PubMed]
68. Han, E.; Tan, M.M.J.; Turk, E.; Sridhar, D.; Leung, G.M.; Shibuya, K.; Asgari, N.; Oh, J.; García-Basteiro, A.L.; Hanefeld, J.; et al. Lessons learnt from easing COVID-19 restrictions: An analysis of countries and regions in Asia Pacific and Europe. *Lancet* **2020**, *396*, 1525–1534. [CrossRef]
69. Sachs, J.D. Comparing COVID-19 control in the Asia-Pacific and North Atlantic regions. *Asian Econ. Pap.* **2021**, *20*, 30–54. [CrossRef]
70. Pearce, N.; Lawlor, D.A.; Brickley, E.B. Comparisons between countries are essential for the control of COVID-19. *Int. J. Epidemiol.* **2020**, *49*, 1059–1062. [CrossRef]

Disclaimer/Publisher's Note: The statements, opinions and data contained in all publications are solely those of the individual author(s) and contributor(s) and not of MDPI and/or the editor(s). MDPI and/or the editor(s) disclaim responsibility for any injury to people or property resulting from any ideas, methods, instructions or products referred to in the content.

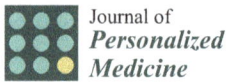

Article

Treatment of Distal Radius Fractures with Bridging External Fixator with Optional Percutaneous K-Wires: What Are the Right Indications for Patient Age, Gender, Dominant Limb and Injury Pattern?

Carlo Biz [1,†], Mariachiara Cerchiaro [1,†], Elisa Belluzzi [1,2,*], Elena Bortolato [3], Alessandro Rossin [1], Antonio Berizzi [1] and Pietro Ruggieri [1]

[1] Orthopedics and Orthopedic Oncology, Department of Surgery, Oncology and Gastroenterology, University of Padova, Via Giustiniani 3, 35128 Padova, Italy
[2] Musculoskeletal Pathology and Oncology Laboratory, Department of Surgery, Oncology and Gastroenterology, University of Padova, Via Giustiniani 3, 35128 Padova, Italy
[3] Department of Statistical Sciences, University of Padova, 35121 Padova, Italy
* Correspondence: elisa.belluzzi@unipd.it; Tel.: +39-049-821-3348
† These authors contributed equally to this work.

Abstract: The aim of this retrospective study was to evaluate the medium-term clinical and functional outcomes of patients with closed, displaced, and unstable, simple or complex, intra- and extra-articular distal radius fractures (DRFs) treated with a bridging external fixator (BEF) and optional K-wires (KWs). AO classification was used to differentiate the injuries radiographically. Clinical-functional outcomes were evaluated using the Patient-Rated Wrist and Hand Evaluation Score (PRWHE Score) and the Quick Disabilities of the Arm Shoulder and Hand Score (QuickDASH). A total of 269 dorsally displaced fractures of 202 female (75%) and 67 male subjects (25%) were included, with a mean follow-up of 58.0 months. Seventy-five patients (28%) were treated by additional KWs. No differences were found comparing the two groups of patients (BEF vs. BEF + KWs) regarding age, sex, and fracture side (dominant vs. non-dominant). PRWHE and QuickDASH scores were lower in the BEF + KWs group compared to the BEF group ($p < 0.0001$ and $p = 0.0007$, respectively). Thus, patients treated with KWs had a better clinical outcome. Beta multivariate regression analysis confirmed that patients of the BEF + KWs group exhibited a better PRWHE score but not a better QuickDASH score. Patients treated by the BEF + KWs with the fracture on the dominant site were characterised by better clinical outcomes. Older patients had a better PRWHE score independently from the treatment. Our findings suggest that the use of BEF for DRFs with optional KWs can be indicated in both young and elderly patients of any gender, independent of limb side and fracture pattern. As the best functional results were achieved in the elderly when KWs were added, the combination of BEF and KWs seems to be mainly indicated for the treatment of DRF, also complex, in the elderly population.

Keywords: distal radius fracture; wrist injury; bridging external fixator; external fixator; K-wires; QuickDASH; PRWHE score

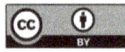

1. Introduction

Distal radius fractures (DRFs) are one of the most common acute events in traumatology, accounting for 17% of all fractures and 1.5–2.5% of access to emergency departments [1]. These fractures are the first in frequency in the general population, followed by fractures of the finger phalanges (11.2%), the metacarpal bones (10.5%), and the proximal femur (8.9%) [2–6]. According to recent studies [7–9], 98.3% of distal forearm fractures have been reported as radius fractures, which may be associated with ulna fractures, and approximately 55% of DRFs are associated with ulnar styloid fractures.

Regarding the trauma mechanism, most fractures are caused by a fall on the hand with the wrist in extension. The pattern and severity of the DRF, as well as the concomitant injuries of the associated disco-ligament structures, depend on the position of the wrist at the moment of impact and the severity of bone fragility. Certainly, the amplitude of this angle influences the location of the fracture [1,10]. For these reasons, the DRFs present a peak in incidence among men under 30 and a peak in women over 60 with osteoporosis [10]. Fractures in young adult patients are usually caused by high-energy trauma, while low-energy dynamics are the most common in geriatric patients [5,11,12]. DRFs are rarely associated to ipsilateral elbow dislocation and instability [13,14].

Depending on the fracture pattern and the AO classification, the therapeutic indication differs [15]. Conservative treatment is preferred mostly for simple undisplaced extra-articular fractures, especially in older low-demand patients and patients who do not require a quick return to work [15–17]. Surgical treatment is necessary in cases of displaced or unstable extra-articular DRFs, simple or complex intra-articular fractures, or in the case of secondary loss of reduction of the fracture [18]. For these, different operative options are available: osteosynthesis with volar or dorsal plates and screws, external wrist fixation, percutaneous fixation with Kirschner wires (KWs), or combinations of the previous two methods. The choice of surgical treatment and the superiority of one method over the others are still debated in the community of orthopaedic surgeons [17,19–21].

Since 2008, external fixation (EF) has become a popular technique in treating unstable DRFs with satisfactory functional results. In this method, some KWs (1.8–2.0 mm) can be added and driven into distal fracture fragments at different angles for improving DRF reduction [22]. Several advantages have been described by using an EF: anatomical reduction of the fracture under fluoroscopic view; increase in reduction by ligamentotaxis, together with the ability to preserve the reduction until the break is healed; simple application of the hardware; minimum operative X-ray exposure; and the reduction of surgical operation time [23]. This type of fixation can be divided into bridging EF and non-bridging EF. In current orthopaedic practice, there are three main types of EF available for adults: F-wrist, Hoffman II Compact, and Pennig Dynamic Wrist Fixator [24].

Comminuted fracture patterns are often difficult to reduce and maintain the reduction over time. Hence, additional KWs are needed as a reduction tool, providing additional stability to the fracture site. To date, only a few studies have focused on the role of optional KWs in EF [12,21], specifically in relation to the bridging fixation technique, and their proper indications is still a source of controversy among orthopaedic surgeons.

The aim of the present study was to investigate and evaluate the medium-term clinical and functional outcomes of patients with closed, displaced, unstable, simple or complex, intra-articular and extra-articular DRFs treated with a bridging external fixator (BEF) and optional percutaneous KWs.

2. Materials and Methods

2.1. Patients

This study was designed as a retrospective, single-centre, comparative, clinical, and functional study, including a consecutive series of Caucasian patients affected by DRFs and treated at our level-I healthcare trauma centre from January 2014 to December 2019 using BEF (Citieffe ST.A.R.90 F4 wrist was the EF available at our institution) with or without additional KWs. At the pre-operative period, all DRFs analysed were classified radiographically according to the AO classification [25].

2.2. Ethics

All subjects participating in this medium-term follow-up study received a thorough explanation of the risks and benefits of inclusion and gave their written informed consent to participate in the study. The approval of the Local Ethics Committee of Padova was obtained (266n/AO/22). The currently reported retrospective cohort study was performed in accordance with the ethical standards of the 1964 Declaration of Helsinki as revised in 2013 and conducted ethically according to the most recent international standards [26].

2.3. Inclusion and Exclusion Criteria

The inclusion criteria were: (1) closed, displaced (fragments not in anatomical alignment with dorsal angulation >15–20 degrees and radial shortening >3 mm [27]) and unstable (comminuted or articular fractures and loss of position following manual reduction [28]) DRFs, extension fractures (Colles's) and articular extension ones treated with BEF and optional KWs; (2) age over 18 at the time of surgery; (3) operation carried out within 72 h after the traumatic event; (4) isolated complete extra-articular or articular fracture of the distal radius; (5) patients who had complete medical records; and (6) patients with a history of physiokinesitherapy for rehabilitation after the removal of BEF.

The exclusion criteria were: (1) open, stable, undisplaced or incomplete DRFs, flexion fractures (Smith) and articular flexion ones; (2) patients who had undergone re-operation or those who had undergone internal osteosynthesis by EF; (3) patients with significant comorbidities (i.e., diabetes, rheumatological, oncological, neurological, or cognitive types, and systemic infection); (4) polytraumatic patients; and (5) patients with previous DRF who were not willing to cooperate with the treatment.

2.4. Surgical Percutaneous Techniques

All operations were performed under brachial plexus regional anaesthesia at our institution by the same trauma team of two surgeons with the patient in supine position on the operating table and maintaining the affected forearm pronated (Figure 1).

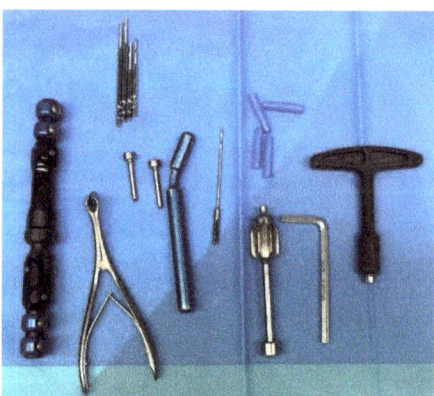

Figure 1. The complete kit of the Bridging External Fixator (BEF) for the wrist by Citieffe.

First, a dorsal incision and blunt dissection were performed at the base of the second metacarpal bone. Two threaded 3 mm bicortical metacarpal pins were introduced into the metacarpal bone at an angle of inclination between 30° and 45° with respect to the horizontal plane (Figure 2).

Second, a longitudinal dorsal incision at the radial border between the middle third and the distal third of the forearm (about 10 cm proximal to the wrist) was performed. After divarication of the subcutis protecting the cutaneous sensory branch of the radial nerve, the bone plane was reached to implant the two bicortical radial pins, respecting the same inclination of 30–45° as the horizontal plane of the forearm. Positioning the BEF body by fixing it to the pin, the fracture reduction was obtained by external manoeuvres under fluoroscopic control, maintaining the wrist in flexion position to stabilise the fracture. Under fluoroscopic control, a percutaneous KW (1.6 mm) was inserted in addition to BEF, from the radial styloid or the dorsum of the radius across the fracture fragments at the surgeon's discretion. The KWs applied were left protruding about 1 cm from the skin and bent so as not to penetrate the soft tissues during the following weeks. After fixation, fluoroscopy was used to check the restoration of volar tilt, radial inclination, ulnar variance, radial height, palmar tilt, articular joint congruency, and external fixator placement (Figure 3).

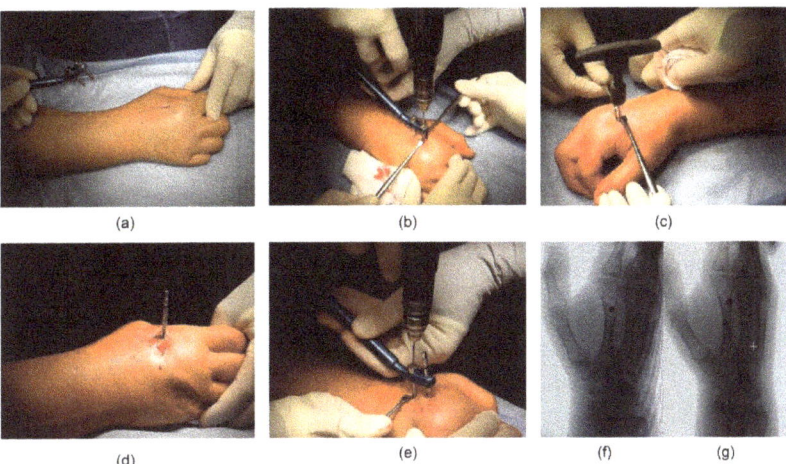

Figure 2. Intra-operative images showing: (**a**) dorsal skin incision at the base of the second metacarpal bone; (**b**–**d**) insertion of the first distal bicortical pin; (**e**) insertion of the second distal cortical pin using the proper tool to maintain the right distance between the pins; antero-posterior (AP) fluoroscopic control of (**f**) the first and (**g**) the second distal pin on the second metacarpal bone.

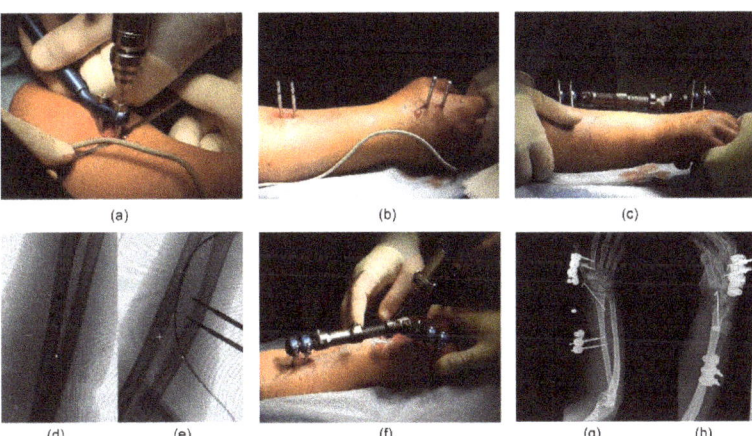

Figure 3. Intra-operative images showing: (**a**) insertion of the pins in the radial diaphysis between the middle third and the distal third of the forearm; (**b**) all pins positioned correctly; (**c**) final application of BEF; (**d**) antero-posterior (AP) and (**e**) latero-lateral (LL) fluoroscopic views of the proximal pins; (**f**) insertion of the KW at the radial styloid level. Post-operative radiographic images: (**g**) AP and (**h**) LL views showing proper reduction and stabilisation of the DRF (AO: 23-C2).

At the end of the surgery, bandages were placed around the pin of the BEF. The external fixator devices and the optional KWs were removed four to five weeks from surgery as an outpatient procedure after radiographic control. The exact timing varied depending on the pin site stability and radiographic evidence of bone fusion or temporary callus bone bridging formation [12,29].

2.5. Post-Operative Protocol of Both Procedures

All patients followed the same post-operative protocol and were followed in the same standardised manner by the senior authors. Active and passive finger mobility was immediately granted. Antero-posterior and lateral X-rays of wrist were taken before the patients were discharged. We recommended an anti-oedemigen therapy (Leucoselect, Lymphaselect, and bromelain: 1 cp/day) for 30 days, starting from the day of the surgery; an analgesic therapy for two weeks with etoricoxib (90 mg, 1 cp/day) in the morning; and if pain persisted, paracetamol/phosphate codeine (1 g, max x3/day) was prescribed. The dressing of the surgical sutures took place seven and fourteen days after surgery, and the removal of sutures on the fourteenth post-operative day. During each scheduled visit, medication at the pin and KW sites was performed until metalwork removal. Post-operative and one- to four-week radiographic checks were performed with subsequent outpatient removal of the body and external wrist fixator pins, including KWs when presented. The remaining wounds at the sites of the pins and KWs were allowed to heal spontaneously.

The physiokinesitherapy process started with the removal of the fixator for an average duration of about three weeks. Active and passive mobilisation was started immediately; resistance activity was granted starting one week after the removal of the fixator. The daily and work activities were gradually resumed, reaching the absence of limitations twelve weeks after the surgery [12] (Figures 4 and 5).

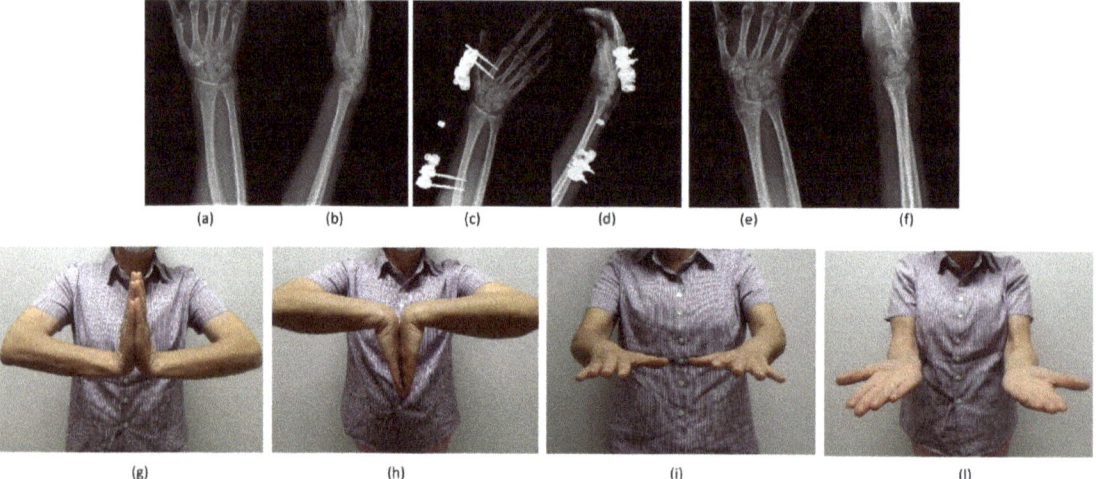

Figure 4. A 69-year-old female patient treated with BEF for an AO 23-B3 DRF. Antero-posterior (AP) and latero-lateral (LL) radiographic images at (**a**,**b**) pre-operative period; (**c**,**d**) immediate post-operative period; (**e**,**f**) at 2-month follow-up. Clinical-functional images showing: (**g**) extension, (**h**) flexion, (**i**) pronation, and (**l**) supination of the operated wrist at last follow-up.

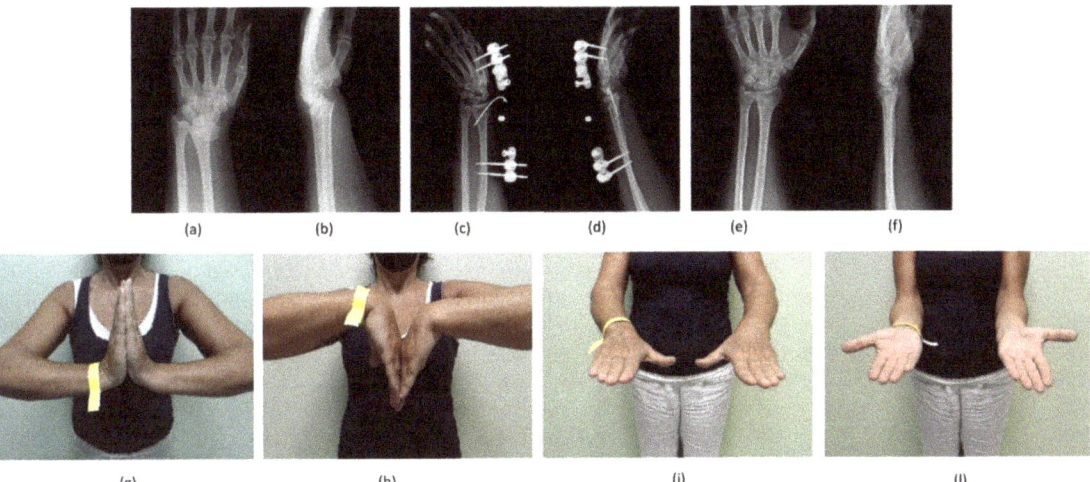

Figure 5. A 58-year-old female patient treated with BEF and an additional KW for an AO 23-C2 DRF. Antero-posterior (AP) and (**b**) latero-lateral (LL) radiographic images at (**a**,**b**) pre-operative period; (**c**,**d**) immediate post-operative period; (**e**,**f**) at 2-month follow-up. Clinical-functional images showing: (**g**) extension, (**h**) flexion, (**i**) pronation, and (**l**) supination of the operated wrist at last follow-up.

2.6. Patient Assessment

Patient characteristics (gender and age at trauma), fracture classification, and dominant side were collected at the baseline. At last follow-up, participants were invited to fill out two different questionnaires for the evaluation of wrist function: the Patient-Rated Wrist Hand Evaluation (PRWHE) and the Quick Disability of the Arm, Shoulder, and Hand (QuickDASH) [30,31]. Both questionnaires are scored from 0 to 100, with higher scores indicating greater disability.

Post-operative complications were recorded and divided between minor and major. Minor complications included wound complications, pain, swelling, and weakness. Major complications included deep infection, chronic infection, non-union, malunion, median nerve-related complaints, and complex regional pain syndrome (CRPS).

According to the surgical treatment, the patients were divided into two groups:

(1) BEF group;
(2) BEF + KWs group.

2.7. Statistical Analysis

Normality of data distribution was verified by conducting the Shapiro–Wilk test. Continuous variables were expressed as mean and standard deviation, while for categorical variables, absolute frequencies and percentage were reported when appropriate. Univariate (Student's *t*-test for unpaired, independent samples, chi-squared test) and multivariate analyses were conducted to assess eventual differences between the two surgical techniques. To understand the effect of the treatment, possible confounders (i.e., age, hand dominance, and sex) were taken into account. It was also noted that the treatment assignment could be influenced by pre-surgery status, which may affect the clinical outcome. Thus, to eliminate the non-randomness of the assignment and to be able to identify the direct effect of treatment on the clinical outcome and that of the covariates, the propensity score (pp) was used. This score measures the treatment dependence on pre-surgery status; hence, conditional on the propensity, the treatment is independent of the pre-surgery status.

The pp was estimated using logistic regression with bias correction [32] and used in the second stage model that also included the treatment and the confounder variables.

For properly modelling the outcome scores, a beta regression model was used that was found to be more suitable in terms of distributional assumptions based on the data. Bias correction techniques implemented in the R package betareg and brglm2 [33] ensured more accurate estimates of standard errors compared to standard maximum likelihoods.

For all analyses, values with p values less than or equal to 0.05 were considered statistically significant. All statistical analyses were performed using R [34].

3. Results

3.1. Patient Data

During a six-year period of enrolment in our institute, 426 patients were treated for dorsally displaced and unstable DRFs with BEF of the wrist. A total of 81 patients were excluded according to the inclusion/exclusion criteria, and a final cohort of 345 patients met the inclusion criteria of this study. Of those, 269 patients were included and completed the follow-up, while 76 patients were excluded (died, were not found, or refused to participate to the study). Therefore, a final cohort of 269 patients was enrolled (Figure 6). All patients were evaluated after an average follow-up of 58 months after surgery (range: 24–87 months).

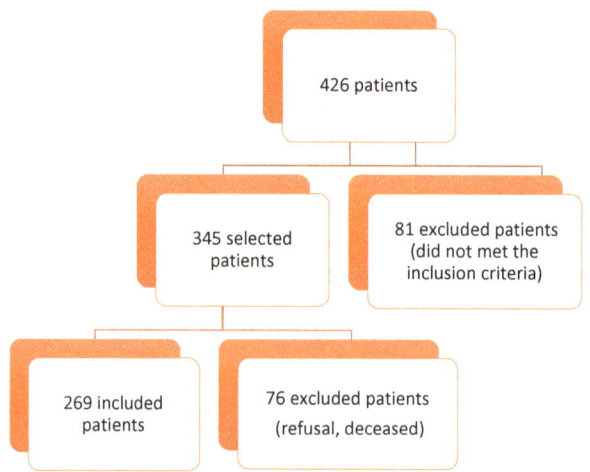

Figure 6. Flowchart of patient selection.

The mean age of the 269 study participants was 65.54 years at the time of surgery (range: 18–94 years); 202 patients were female (75%) and 67 were male (25%). Fractures of the dominant side occurred in 106 patients (39.4%), while the remaining fractures were on the non-dominant side (163 patients, 60.6%). The mean PHRWE was 12.18 ± 15.75 and mean QuickDASH was 13.13 ± 15.86 of the overall cohort at the follow-up. Fractures were classified using the AO classification system (Table 1).

Considering the overall cohort, no differences between PRWHE and AO classification ($p = 0.40$) or gender ($p = 0.35$) were observed. Likewise, no differences between QuickDASH and AO classification ($p = 0.43$) or gender ($p = 0.21$) were found. A weak negative correlation was found between clinical scores and age (PRWHE: $r = -0.21$; $p < 0.001$ and QuickDASH: $r = -0.22$; $p < 0.001$). Of the 266 cases, 75 (28%) were treated by associating KWs to the BEF. No differences were found comparing the two groups of patients (BEF vs. BEF + KWs) regarding age, sex, and fracture side (dominant vs. non-dominant). PRWHE and QuickDASH scores were lower in BEF + KWs group compared to BEF, indicating that patients with KWs have a better clinical outcome ($p < 0.0001$ and $p = 0.0007$, respectively) (Table 2).

Table 1. Overall cohort characteristics.

Variable	Patients (n = 269)
Age	65.55 ± 15.27
Sex	
Female	202 (75.1%)
Male	67 (24.9%)
PRWHE	12.18 ± 15.75
QuickDASH	13.13 ± 15.86
Side	
Dominant	106 (39.4%)
Non-dominant	163 (60.6%)
AO classification (23)	
A2	48 (17.8%)
A3	39 (14.5%)
B1	2 (0.7%)
B3	1 (0.4%)
C1	50 (18.6%)
C2	82 (30.5%)
C3	47 (17.5%)

Table 2. Comparison between BEF and BEF + KWs groups.

Variable	BEF (194 Patients)	BEF + KWs (75 Patients)	p-Value
Age	65.83 ± 15.24	64.81 ± 15.44	0.59
Sex			
Female	148 (76.3%)	54 (72%)	0.57
Male	46 (23.7%)	21 (28%)	
PRWHE	14.59 ± 17.04	5.88 ± 9.20	<0.001
QuickDASH	15.30 ± 17.10	7.50 ± 10.16	<0.001
Side			
Dominant	79 (40.7%)	27 (36%)	0.57
Non-dominant	115 (59.3%)	48 (64%)	
AO classification (23)			
A2	41 (21.1%)	7 (9.3%)	
A3	30 (15.5%)	9 (12.0%)	
B1	0 (0%)	2 (2.7%)	
B3	1 (0.5%)	0 (0%)	0.007
C1	40 (20.6%)	10 (13.3%)	
C2	53 (27.3%)	29 (38.7%)	
C3	29 (14.9%)	18 (24.0%)	

3.2. Complications

Minor complications were recorded in 70 patients (26%). Discomfort due to the presence of the BEF was reported by 23 patients. Twenty patients had superficial pin infections, which were successfully treated with oral antibiotics. Complex regional pain syndrome (CRPS) occurred in six patients. Radial nerve injury was found in four patients. Radial shortening was recorded in five patients. Tendon irritation occurred in 12 patients.

3.3. Multivariate Analysis

With the beta multivariate regression analysis, it was confirmed that patients of the BEF + KWs groups exhibited a better PRWHE score; however, no influence was reported with QuickDASH. Patients of the BEF + KWs with the fracture on the dominant site were characterised by a better clinical outcome (both PRWHE and QuickDASH). Older patients had a better PRWHE score independently from the treatment. No influence was observed regarding fracture type and fracture type associated with treatment type (Tables 3 and 4).

Table 3. Beta multivariate regression analysis of the impact of the different variables on PRWHE score.

Variable	Estimate	Standard Error	Z Value	p-Value
Intercept	−0.377	0.436	−0.866	0.386
pp	−0.976	1.739	−0.561	0.575
BEF + KWs	−0.385	0.165	−2.334	0.020
Dominant side	0.275	0.133	2.065	0.039
Age	−0.018	0.004	−4.004	<0.001
23-A3	−0.310	0.254	−1.224	0.220
23-B	−0.173	0.955	−0.181	0.856
23-C1	−0.002	0.214	−0.010	0.992
23-C2	0.006	0.386	0.017	0.986
23-C3	0.182	0.439	0.416	0.677
BEF + KWs and dominant side	−0.410	0.266	−1.545	0.122
Phi coefficients				
Intercept	0.186	0439	0.425	0.671
Age	0.014	0.006	2.551	0.011
pp	2.168	0.888	2.441	0.015

Table 4. Beta multivariate regression analysis of the impact of the different variables on QuickDASH score.

Variable	Estimate	Standard Error	Z Value	p-Value
Intercept	−0.378	0.433	−0.874	0.382
pp	0.211	1.735	0.122	0.903
BEF + KWs	−0.249	0.165	−1.516	0.129
Dominant side	0.354	0.133	2.664	0.008
Age	−0.020	0.004	−4.544	<0.001
23-A3	−0.362	0.251	−1.447	0.148
23-B	−0.616	0.960	−0.641	0.521
23-C1	−0.156	0.211	−0.740	0.459
23-C2	−0.263	0.385	−0.682	0.495
23-C3	−0.120	0.438	−0.273	0.785
BEF + KWs and dominant side	−0.468	0.264	−1.775	0.076
Phi coefficients				
Intercept	−0.012	0.430	−0.029	0.977
Age	1.546	0.876	1.764	0.078
pp	0.020	0.006	3.586	<0.001

In order to interpret the effect sizes estimated by the model, some examples of predicted scores could be compared that differ for a change of variable associated to a significant coefficient in the model. Taking as a reference group the one with median characteristics for quantitative variables (propensity score equal to 0.27, age 68), fracture of type A2, no KWs, and non-dominant side, the estimated scores were 13.29 for PRWHE and 15.31 for QuickDASH. For the group with the same characteristics but dominant side, the scores became 16.79 and 20.48, respectively. Changing the treatment group from BEF to BEF + K-wires, the scores within the reference group dropped from 13.29 to 9.44 (PRWHE) and from 15.31 to 12.34 (QuickDASH) for the non-dominant side, and from 16.79 to 8.34 (PRWHE) and from 20.48 to 11.16 (QuickDASH) for the dominant side.

Regarding age, there is a progressive decrease of the scores as the age of patients increases, keeping all of the other characteristics fixed. The predicted range is between 10.98 for 20-year-old individuals and 26.80 for 80-year-old individuals (PRWHE) and from 12.34 for 20-years-olds to 32.52 for 80-year-olds (QuickDASH).

4. Discussion

DRFs are common orthopaedic injuries, occurring within 3 cm of the distal part of the radius, with a bimodal age distribution (a peak in incidence among men under 30 and a peak in women over 60 with osteoporosis). The two main trauma mechanisms are high-energy trauma and low-energy falls, respectively [5,7].

Management of DRFs includes closed reduction and casting, closed reduction and percutaneous fixation, and open reduction internal fixation with volar or dorsal plating [35]. Immobilisation with wrist casts is the conservative solution reserved for simple displaced or minimally displaced extra-articular fractures, especially if the patient does not require a quick return to work [16,36,37]. About 35% of total DRFs require surgery. Unstable extra-articular and intra-articular fractures of the distal epiphysis of the radius usually require surgical treatment [36,38]. For these injuries, however, there is still no agreement on what the optimal treatment is in relation to age, gender, dominant limb, and fracture pattern.

In our study, we compared the scores of two questionnaires for the evaluation of functional outcomes in patients with DRFs treated with a BEF and optional KWs divided into categories on the basis of age, type of treatment, pattern fracture, gender, and limb dominance. Only closed, displaced, and unstable extension fractures (Colles's) and articular extension fractures were included, because flexion fractures (Smith) and articular flexion fractures were treated by plate osteosynthesis according to our institutional wrist trauma protocol. The most important finding of our analysis was that no differences between PRWHE and AO classification ($p = 0.40$) or gender ($p = 0.35$) were observed in our overall cohort at the mean follow-up of 58 months. Likewise, no differences between QuickDASH and AO classification ($p = 0.43$) or gender ($p = 0.21$) were found.

Although the comparison of EF versus volar plates and screws (VLP) in unstable DRF was not the objective of this study, a meta-analysis comparing both techniques concluded that cases treated with a VLP could obtain better functional outcomes [39]. In contrast, a recent meta-analysis and systematic review showed that patients treated with VLP had a lower DASH score and VAS score, and no significant differences in radiographic outcomes were observed even if VLP had a lower complication rate than that of EF [29]. Another study reported that VLP fixation resulted in faster recovery of function compared to EF, but no functional advantage was demonstrated at two years' short follow-up [40]. Furthermore, patients undergoing DRF surgery with open reduction and internal fixation (ORIF) have a higher risk of wound infection and tendonitis [41].

Hence, the results from the literature suggest that surgery yields statistically but not clinically better functional outcomes at one-year follow-up [42]. Treatment with VLP might benefit patients who have the need to gain the previous level of activity in a short period of time. However, it deserves mention that the current literature does not provide an actual cut-off for age, fracture malalignment, or other specific factors.

Regarding the population age, some authors have underlined a variety of differences in demographic factors, considering the EF more commonly indicated in younger, male patients who are more likely to have higher energy trauma and more significant distal radius comminution [43]. On the contrary, in our cohort, a weak negative correlation was found between clinical scores and age (PRWHE: $r = -0.21$; $p < 0.001$ and QuickDASH: $r = -0.22$; $p < 0.001$). Specifically, the difference in terms of functional results between EF in the elderly and in the younger patients was not statistically significant, although young people require a greater degree of functionality than the elderly and a better possible reduction in fracture, which is not always anatomically obtainable by BEF. Furthermore, the general evaluation of the results between AO 23A and AO 23C fracture pattern did not show statistical significance among young and elderly patients. These findings can be justified by the fact that the functional-clinical outcomes can be perceived subjectively in different ways for the different injury patterns by the two populations.

Certainly, BEF is not always able to guarantee the alignment of the fracture fragments and the stability of the reduction, especially in cases of articular or metaphyseal involvement or severe periarticular injury [44]. For these reasons, in some cases, we preferred associated percutaneous KWs, which were useful to reduce and stabilise the fractures during surgery, and they contributed to achieving good functional outcomes at medium-term follow-up, which are shown in the BEF + KWs group. Rectenwald et al. [45] also demonstrated how the association of EF and KWs not only allows improvement of stability but also maintains the reduction obtained with simple EF until bone callus formation.

To date, only a few studies have focused on the role of additional KWs in EF [12]. Among the 269 cases included in our study, 75 (28%) were treated by associating percutaneous synthesis with KWs to the BEF. No differences were found comparing the two groups of patients (BEF vs. BEF + KWs) regarding age, sex, and fracture side (dominant vs. non-dominant), and all patients of both groups were able to resume normal daily life activities after the operation. However, PRWHE and QuickDASH scores were lower in the BEF + KWs groups compared to EF ($p < 0.0001$ and $p = 0.0007$, respectively), indicating that patients with KWs had a better clinical outcome. Patients of the BEF group with a fracture on the dominant site had a worse clinical outcome (higher scores) than those with the fracture on the non-dominant side. The opposite occurred in the BEF + KWs group: patients with the fracture on the dominant side had better clinical outcomes. In other words, the predicted scores for patients with the dominant side injured are better (lower) for the patients treated with BEF + KWs than with the BEF alone. In the group with the non-dominant side injured, the clinical outcome is still better for those treated with BEF + KWs with respect to those treated with BEF only, even if the difference is less evident. It should be noted that the scores obtained are very good. Importantly, beta multivariate regression analysis confirmed that the BEF + KWs group exhibited a better PRWHE score; however, no influence was reported with QuickDASH. However, patients of the BEF + KWs with the fracture on the dominant site were characterised by a better clinical outcome (both PRWHE and QuickDASH). Older patients had better PRWHE scores independently of the treatment, probably because of low demand. No influence was observed regarding fracture type and fracture type associated with treatment type. Our clinical functional results are in line with those of another scientific report: Fu et al. [46] demonstrated how the combination of BEF and KWs leads to better clinical-functional results than simple BEF.

In the literature, there is agreement in the definition of what is the least clinically relevant difference between mean functional scores: according to the meta-analyses of Li-hai et al. (2015) [47] and Walenkamp et al. [48] and the study of Gummesson et al. [49], the minimal score difference describing a clinically significant difference after two upper limb surgical treatments is a mean difference of 10 points. In our study, we recorded significant differences between means greater than 10 points (or approximately 10 points), in agreement with the literature.

Wrist EF has many advantages in the treatment of DRFs. First, it scarcely affects the blood supply around the fracture ends, which is conducive to recanalisation of bone vessels and creates a good fracture-healing environment. Second, non-cross-joint fixation allows normal movement of the wrist, diminishes stiffness, stimulates cartilage repair, decreases osteopenia of the distal fragment and reduces fear among patients [41].

In our groups, fractures of the dominant side occurred in 106 patients (39.4%), while the remaining fractures were on the non-dominant side (163 patients, 60.6%). The analysis of the data relative to the dominant limb is interesting as it did not show major functional deficits in daily activities with respect to the non-dominant limb between the two procedure groups. Hence, good results were recorded for the dominant limb independent of the procedure used. Our results relating to the proper use of BEF, with optional KWs, in DRFs in relation to patient age, gender, dominant limb, and injury pattern do not find comparable precedents in the literature.

Given the known epidemiological difference in the prevalence of DRFs, no significant differences were found in the outcomes of patients of different genders, which is simple evidence that gender-specific factor-related activities are not involved in the subjectivity of filling out the outcome questionnaires. These results agree with the results of other scientific reports presented in literature: the study by Lee et al. [50] did not identify statistical significance for the gender variable in terms of post-operative functional results; Synn et al. [17] found no influence of patient gender.

In the literature, EF use for the treatment of DRF is associated with a 24% to 62% complication rate, most of which includes superficial pin site infection, malunion, and loss of radiocarpal and digital motion [51–56]. Specifically, Weber and Szabo reported a 62% complication rate associated with EF, most commonly loose pins, pin tract infection, and malreduction [55].

Normally, pin tract infections range between 0 and 27% [55,57–59]. However, Anderson et al. reported 37.5% pin tract infection; all infections were resolved with antibiotics [52]. Raskin and Melone reported no pin tract infections in their study [60]. They attribute this to their method of pin site care. Carpal tunnel syndrome (4.3% non-operative, 1.9% surgery) has been reported more commonly in non-operatively treated patients and in those treated by VLP [42]. In our study, the minor complications registered (superficial pin infection, discomfort from external hardware, and tendon irritation) were all resolved in a short time, and none affected the clinical functional outcomes at last follow-up. For these reasons, as trauma surgeons, we think these must be considered part of the surgical procedure and the post-operative period rather than sequalae of the treatment method. On the contrary, the few major complications reported—carpal tunnel syndrome, CRPS, radial nerve injury, and radial shortening—impacted medium-term results. We did not find malunion or nonunion, contrary to what is reported in the study of Anderson at al. [52], where their incidence was surprisingly high (12.5%).

Over-distraction can cause increased pressure in the carpal tunnel, according to Gelberman et al. [61]. To avoid this, Hertel and Ballmer suggest first obtaining preliminary reduction with over-distraction and then stabilising the fracture with crossed KWs, followed by reduction of distraction to neutral length and position [62]. The incidence of superficial radial nerve irritation could be largely dependent on the surgeon's technique of pin placement. Using an open technique, the superficial branch of the radial nerve can be protected.

Discomfort from external hardware, finger stiffness, loss of reduction, and complex regional pain syndrome are other complications [54,55,63–67]. Patients who receive an external fixator have reported more discomfort and reduced health-related quality of life when compared with internal fixation [53].

Some potential limitations may have influenced the results of our study: (i) its retrospective nature and the different sizes among BEF and BEF + KWs (192 vs. 72); (ii) the wide range of follow-up, from a minimum of 24 months after surgery to a maximum of 87 months; (iii) the lack of objective evaluation of range of motion in the follow-up of our patients, as well as the lack of radiographic evaluations in the study. This could have affected our clinical-functional outcomes at medium-term follow-up, as they were based only on the subjectivity of the patients, without a radiographic correlation. Another weakness is the lack of a control group treated by ORIF, which would be useful to compare the results of our technique. Finally, it is necessary to underline that the AO fracture classification used for our analysis was based on standard radiographs, as computed tomography was performed only in the cases of intraarticular injuries with multiple fragments, according to our institutional protocol.

Nevertheless, to the best of our knowledge, this is the first single-centre study reporting functional clinical outcomes of DRFs at medium-term follow-up and including beta multivariate regression analysis on a large patient cohort compared to previous published studies on the same topic [12,46,68–70]. Further, all patients enrolled were operated on by the same trauma surgeons and followed according to a standardised institutional post-operative protocol, reducing confounding bias. Importantly, the functional limitations of treated wrists were evaluated using two validated questionnaires whose reliability, validity, and specificity have been confirmed by several studies [71]: the PRWHE Score, a specific tool only for DRFs assessment, and the QuickDASH, a widespread method for upper limb evaluation.

Future randomised controlled clinical trials comparing the BEF procedure with optional KWs to other operative methods are necessary to better define optimal indications for the treatment of unstable DRFs in both young and elderly patients and provide further useful information in relation to fracture pattern.

5. Conclusions

The medium-term functional-clinical outcomes of this retrospective study and their beta multivariate analysis suggest that the use of BEF with optional KWs for the treatment of unstable DRFs can be indicated in both young and elderly patients of any gender, independent of limb side and fracture pattern. Nevertheless, as the best functional results were achieved in the elderly when KWs were added to stabilise and maintain the fracture reduction, in particular of the dominant side, the combination of BEF and KWs seems to be mainly indicated for the treatment of DRF, also complex, in the elderly population.

Author Contributions: Conceptualization, C.B. and P.R.; methodology, C.B., M.C., and E.B. (Elisa Belluzzi); validation, C.B., M.C., E.B. (Elisa Belluzzi), and A.B.; formal analysis, E.B. (Elena Bortolato) and E.B. (Elisa Belluzzi); investigation, M.C. and A.R.; resources, C.B., A.B., and P.R.; data curation, C.B. and E.B. (Elisa Belluzzi); writing—original draft preparation, C.B., M.C., and E.B. (Elisa Belluzzi); writing—review and editing, C.B., M.C., E.B. (Elena Bortolato), and E.B. (Elisa Belluzzi); visualization, E.B. (Elisa Belluzzi) and A.R.; supervision, P.R.; project administration, C.B. and E.B. (Elisa Belluzzi). All authors have read and agreed to the published version of the manuscript.

Funding: This research received no external funding.

Institutional Review Board Statement: The study was conducted in accordance with the Declaration of Helsinki and approved by the Ethics Committee of University-Hospital of Padova (protocol code 266n/AO/22 and 30 June 2022).

Informed Consent Statement: Informed consent was obtained from all subjects involved in the study.

Data Availability Statement: The dataset supporting the conclusions of this review is available upon request to the corresponding author.

Conflicts of Interest: The authors declare no conflict of interest.

References

1. Nellans, K.W.; Kowalski, E.; Chung, K.C. The epidemiology of distal radius fractures. *Hand Clin.* **2012**, *28*, 113–125. [CrossRef] [PubMed]
2. Singer, B.R.; McLauchlan, G.J.; Robinson, C.M.; Christie, J. Epidemiology of fractures in 15,000 adults: The influence of age and gender. *J. Bone Joint Surg. Br.* **1998**, *80*, 243–248. [CrossRef] [PubMed]
3. Schuit, S.C.; van der Klift, M.; Weel, A.E.; de Laet, C.E.; Burger, H.; Seeman, E.; Hofman, A.; Uitterlinden, A.G.; van Leeuwen, J.P.; Pols, H.A. Fracture incidence and association with bone mineral density in elderly men and women: The Rotterdam Study. *Bone* **2004**, *34*, 195–202. [CrossRef]
4. Court-Brown, C.M.; Caesar, B. Epidemiology of adult fractures: A review. *Injury* **2006**, *37*, 691–697. [CrossRef] [PubMed]
5. Meena, S.; Sharma, P.; Sambharia, A.K.; Dawar, A. Fractures of Distal Radius: An Overview. *J. Fam. Med. Prim. Care* **2014**, *3*, 325–332. [CrossRef]
6. Biz, C.; Tagliapietra, J.; Zonta, F.; Belluzzi, E.; Bragazzi, N.L.; Ruggieri, P. Predictors of early failure of the cannulated screw system in patients, 65 years and older, with non-displaced femoral neck fractures. *Aging Clin. Exp. Res.* **2020**, *32*, 505–513. [CrossRef] [PubMed]
7. Krämer, S.; Meyer, H.; O'Loughlin, P.F.; Vaske, B.; Krettek, C.; Gaulke, R. The incidence of ulnocarpal complaints after distal radial fracture in relation to the fracture of the ulnar styloid. *J. Hand Surg. (Eur. Vol.)* **2012**, *38*, 710–717. [CrossRef]
8. May, M.M.; Lawton, J.N.; Blazar, P.E. Ulnar styloid fractures associated with distal radius fractures: Incidence and implications for distal radioulnar joint instability. *J. Hand Surg.* **2002**, *27*, 965–971. [CrossRef] [PubMed]
9. Iacobellis, C.; Biz, C. Plating in diaphyseal fractures of the forearm. *Acta Biomed.* **2014**, *84*, 202–211.
10. MacIntyre, N.J.; Dewan, N. Epidemiology of distal radius fractures and factors predicting risk and prognosis. *J. Hand Ther.* **2016**, *29*, 136–145. [CrossRef]

11. Levin, L.S.; Rozell, J.C.; Pulos, N. Distal Radius Fractures in the Elderly. *JAAOS J. Am. Acad. Orthop. Surg.* **2017**, *25*, 179–187. [CrossRef] [PubMed]
12. Cheng, P.; Wu, F.; Chen, H.; Jiang, C.; Wang, T.; Han, P.; Chai, Y. Early hybrid nonbridging external fixation of unstable distal radius fractures in patients aged ≥50 years. *J. Int. Med. Res.* **2020**, *48*, 0300060519879562. [CrossRef] [PubMed]
13. Bäcker, H.C.; Thiele, K.; Wu, C.H.; Moroder, P.; Stöckle, U.; Braun, K.F. Distal Radius Fracture with Ipsilateral Elbow Dislocation: A Rare but Challenging Injury. *J. Pers. Med.* **2022**, *12*, 1097. [CrossRef] [PubMed]
14. Biz, C.; Crimì, A.; Belluzzi, E.; Maschio, N.; Baracco, R.; Volpin, A.; Ruggieri, P. Conservative Versus Surgical Management of Elbow Medial Ulnar Collateral Ligament Injury: A Systematic Review. *Orthop. Surg.* **2019**, *11*, 974–984. [CrossRef]
15. Buckley, R.E. *AO Principles of Fracture Management*; Thieme Medical Publishers: New York, NY, USA, 2018. [CrossRef]
16. Young, B.T.; Rayan, G.M. Outcome following nonoperative treatment of displaced distal radius fractures in low-demand patients older than 60 years. *J. Hand Surg.* **2000**, *25*, 19–28. [CrossRef]
17. Synn, A.J.; Makhni, E.C.; Makhni, M.C.; Rozental, T.D.; Day, C.S. Distal Radius Fractures in Older Patients: Is Anatomic Reduction Necessary? *Clin. Orthop. Relat. Res.* **2009**, *467*, 1612–1620. [CrossRef]
18. Obert, L.; Rey, P.B.; Uhring, J.; Gasse, N.; Rochet, S.; Lepage, D.; Serre, A.; Garbuio, P. Fixation of distal radius fractures in adults: A review. *Orthop. Traumatol. Surg. Res.* **2013**, *99*, 216–234. [CrossRef]
19. Handoll, H.H.G.; Madhok, R. From evidence to best practice in the management of fractures of the distal radius in adults: Working towards a research agenda. *BMC Musculoskelet. Disord.* **2003**, *4*, 27. [CrossRef]
20. Padegimas, E.M.; Ilyas, A.M. Distal radius fractures: Emergency department evaluation and management. *Orthop. Clin. N. Am.* **2015**, *46*, 259–270. [CrossRef]
21. Mellstrand Navarro, C.; Ahrengart, L.; Törnqvist, H.; Ponzer, S. Volar Locking Plate or External Fixation with Optional Addition of K-Wires for Dorsally Displaced Distal Radius Fractures: A Randomized Controlled Study. *J. Orthop. Trauma* **2016**, *30*, 217–224. [CrossRef]
22. Liu, Y.; Bai, Y.M. Efficacy of non-bridging external fixation in treating distal radius fractures. *Orthop. Surg.* **2020**, *12*, 776–783. [CrossRef] [PubMed]
23. Sharma, A.; Pathak, S.; Sandhu, H.; Bagtharia, P.; Kumar, N.; Bajwa, R.S.; Pruthi, V.; Chawla, J.S. Prospective randomized study comparing the external fixator and volar locking plate in intraarticular distal radius fractures: Which is better? *Cureus* **2020**, *12*, e6849. [CrossRef]
24. Li, J.; Rai, S.; Tang, X.; Ze, R.; Liu, R.; Hong, P. Fixation of delayed distal radial fracture involving metaphyseal diaphyseal junction in adolescents: A comparative study of crossed Kirschner-wiring and non-bridging external fixator. *BMC Musculoskelet. Disord.* **2020**, *21*, 365. [CrossRef] [PubMed]
25. Marsh, J.L.; Slongo, T.F.; Agel, J.; Broderick, J.S.; Creevey, W.; DeCoster, T.A.; Prokuski, L.; Sirkin, M.S.; Ziran, B.; Henley, B.; et al. Fracture and dislocation classification compendium—2007: Orthopaedic Trauma Association classification, database and outcomes committee. *J. Orthop. Trauma* **2007**, *21*, S1–S133. [CrossRef] [PubMed]
26. Padulo, J.; Oliva, F.; Frizziero, A.; Maffulli, N. Basic principles and recommendations in clinical and field science research. *Muscles Ligaments Tendons J.* **2013**, *3*, 250–252.
27. Leixnering, M.; Rosenauer, R.; Pezzei, C.; Jurkowitsch, J.; Beer, T.; Keuchel, T.; Simon, D.; Hausner, T.; Quadlbauer, S. Indications, surgical approach, reduction, and stabilization techniques of distal radius fractures. *Arch. Orthop. Trauma Surg.* **2020**, *140*, 611–621. [CrossRef]
28. Walenkamp, M.M.; Vos, L.M.; Strackee, S.D.; Goslings, J.C.; Schep, N.W. The Unstable Distal Radius Fracture-How Do We Define It? A Systematic Review. *J. Wrist Surg.* **2015**, *4*, 307–316. [CrossRef]
29. Gou, Q.; Xiong, X.; Cao, D.; He, Y.; Li, X. Volar locking plate versus external fixation for unstable distal radius fractures: A systematic review and meta-analysis based on randomized controlled trials. *BMC Musculoskelet. Disord.* **2021**, *22*, 433. [CrossRef]
30. Fairplay, T.; Atzei, A.; Corradi, M.; Luchetti, R.; Cozzolino, R.; Schoenhuber, R. Cross-cultural adaptation and validation of the Italian version of the patient-rated wrist/hand evaluation questionnaire. *J. Hand Surg. (Eur. Vol.)* **2012**, *37*, 863–870. [CrossRef]
31. Beaton, D.E.; Wright, J.G.; Katz, J.N. Development of the QuickDASH: Comparison of three item-reduction approaches. *J. Bone Jt. Surgery. Am. Vol.* **2005**, *87*, 1038–1046. [CrossRef]
32. Firth, D. Bias reduction of maximum likelihood estimates. *Biometrika* **1993**, *80*, 27–38. [CrossRef]
33. Kosmidis, I. brglm2: Bias Reduction in Generalized Linear Models. Available online: https://CRAN.R-project.org/package=brglm2 (accessed on 28 June 2022).
34. R Core Team. *R: A Language and Environment for Statistical Computing*; R Foundation for Statistical Computing: Vienna, Austria, 2014.
35. Chhabra, A.B.; Yildirim, B. Adult Distal Radius Fracture Management. *JAAOS J. Am. Acad. Orthop. Surg.* **2021**, *29*, e1105–e1116. [CrossRef]
36. Rüedi, T.P.; Murphy, W.M.; Colton, C.L.; Fackelman, G.E.; Harder, Y. *AO Principles of Fracture Management*; Thieme: Stuttgart, Germany, 2000.
37. Patterson, M. Apley's Concise System of Orthopaedics and Fractures 3rd edn). *Ann. R. Coll. Surg. Engl.* **2006**, *88*, 425–426. [CrossRef]
38. Chen, N.C.; Jupiter, J.B. Management of distal radial fractures. *J. Bone Jt. Surgery. Am. Vol.* **2007**, *89*, 2051–2062. [CrossRef]

39. Walenkamp, M.M.; Bentohami, A.; Beerekamp, M.S.; Peters, R.W.; van der Heiden, R.; Goslings, J.C.; Schep, N.W. Functional outcome in patients with unstable distal radius fractures, volar locking plate versus external fixation: A meta-analysis. *Strateg. Trauma Limb Reconstr.* **2013**, *8*, 67–75. [CrossRef]
40. Hammer, O.L.; Clementsen, S.; Hast, J.; Šaltytė Benth, J.; Madsen, J.E.; Randsborg, P.H. Volar Locking Plates Versus Augmented External Fixation of Intra-Articular Distal Radial Fractures: Functional Results from a Randomized Controlled Trial. *J. Bone Jt. Surgery. Am. Vol.* **2019**, *101*, 311–321. [CrossRef]
41. Xie, M.; Cao, Y.; Cai, X.; Shao, Z.; Nie, K.; Xiong, L. The Effect of a PEEK Material-Based External Fixator in the Treatment of Distal Radius Fractures with Non-Transarticular External Fixation. *Orthop. Surg.* **2021**, *13*, 90–97. [CrossRef]
42. Luokkala, T.; Laitinen, M.K.; Hevonkorpi, T.P.; Raittio, L.; Mattila, V.M.; Launonen, A.P. Distal radius fractures in the elderly population. *EFORT Open Rev.* **2020**, *5*, 361–370. [CrossRef]
43. Vakhshori, V.; Rounds, A.D.; Heckmann, N.; Azad, A.; Intravia, J.M.; Rosario, S.; Stevanovic, M.; Ghiassi, A. The Declining Use of Wrist-Spanning External Fixators. *Hand (N Y)* **2020**, *15*, 255–263. [CrossRef]
44. Tang, J.B. Distal Radius Fracture: Diagnosis, Treatment, and Controversies. *Clin. Plast. Surg.* **2014**, *41*, 481–499. [CrossRef]
45. Rectenwald, J.P.; Bentley, K.A.; Murray, P.M.; Saha, S. Strain as a Function of Time in Extrinsic Wrist Ligaments Tensioned Through External Fixation. *Hand (N Y)* **2018**, *13*, 60–64. [CrossRef]
46. Fu, Y.C.; Chien, S.H.; Huang, P.J.; Chen, S.K.; Tien, Y.C.; Lin, G.T.; Wang, G.J. Use of an external fixation combined with the buttress-maintain pinning method in treating comminuted distal radius fractures in osteoporotic patients. *J. Trauma* **2006**, *60*, 330–333. [CrossRef]
47. Zhang, L.; Wang, Y.; Mao, Z.; Zhang, L.; Li, H.; Yan, H.; Liu, X.; Tang, P. Volar locking plate versus external fixation for the treatment of unstable distal radial fractures: A meta-analysis of randomized controlled trials. *J. Surg. Res.* **2015**, *193*, 324–333. [CrossRef]
48. Walenkamp, M.M.J.; Mulders, M.A.M.; Goslings, J.C.; Westert, G.P.; Schep, N.W.L. Analysis of variation in the surgical treatment of patients with distal radial fractures in the Netherlands. *J. Hand Surg. Eur. Vol.* **2017**, *42*, 39–44. [CrossRef]
49. Gummesson, C.; Atroshi, I.; Ekdahl, C. The disabilities of the arm, shoulder and hand (DASH) outcome questionnaire: Longitudinal construct validity and measuring self-rated health change after surgery. *BMC Musculoskelet. Disord.* **2003**, *4*, 11. [CrossRef]
50. Lee, S.J.; Park, J.W.; Kang, B.J.; Lee, J.I. Clinical and radiologic factors affecting functional outcomes after volar locking plate fixation of dorsal angulated distal radius fractures. *J. Orthop. Sci. Off. J. Jpn. Orthop. Assoc.* **2016**, *21*, 619–624. [CrossRef]
51. Capo, J.T.; Rossy, W.; Henry, P.; Maurer, R.J.; Naidu, S.; Chen, L. External fixation of distal radius fractures: Effect of distraction and duration. *J. Hand Surg.* **2009**, *34*, 1605–1611. [CrossRef]
52. Anderson, J.T.; Lucas, G.L.; Buhr, B.R. Complications of treating distal radius fractures with external fixation: A community experience. *Iowa Orthop. J.* **2004**, *24*, 53–59.
53. Ma, C.; Deng, Q.; Pu, H.; Cheng, X.; Kan, Y.; Yang, J.; Yusufu, A.; Cao, L. External fixation is more suitable for intra-articular fractures of the distal radius in elderly patients. *Bone Res.* **2016**, *4*, 16017. [CrossRef]
54. Sanders, R.A.; Keppel, F.L.; Waldrop, J.I. External fixation of distal radial fractures: Results and complications. *J. Hand Surg.* **1991**, *16*, 385–391. [CrossRef]
55. Weber, S.C.; Szabo, R.M. Severely comminuted distal radial fracture as an unsolved problem: Complications associated with external fixation and pins and plaster techniques. *J. Hand Surg.* **1986**, *11*, 157–165. [CrossRef]
56. Xie, X.; Xie, X.; Qin, H.; Shen, L.; Zhang, C. Comparison of internal and external fixation of distal radius fractures. *Acta Orthop.* **2013**, *84*, 286–291. [CrossRef]
57. Edwards, G.S., Jr. Intra-articular fractures of the distal part of the radius treated with the small AO external fixator. *J. Bone Jt. Surgery. Am. Vol.* **1991**, *73*, 1241–1250. [CrossRef]
58. Dienst, M.; Wozasek, G.E.; Seligson, D. Dynamic external fixation for distal radius fractures. *Clin. Orthop. Relat. Res.* **1997**, *338*, 160–171. [CrossRef]
59. Horesh, Z.; Volpin, G.; Hoerer, D.; Stein, H. The surgical treatment of severe comminuted intraarticular fractures of the distal radius with the small AO external fixation device. A prospective three-and-one-half-year follow-up study. *Clin. Orthop. Relat. Res.* **1991**, *263*, 147–153. [CrossRef]
60. Raskin, K.B.; Melone, C.P., Jr. Unstable articular fractures of the distal radius. Comparative techniques of ligamentotaxis. *Orthop. Clin. N. Am.* **1993**, *24*, 275–286. [CrossRef]
61. Gelberman, R.H.; Szabo, R.M.; Mortensen, W.W. Carpal tunnel pressures and wrist position in patients with colles' fractures. *J. Trauma* **1984**, *24*, 747–749. [CrossRef]
62. Hertel, R.; Ballmer, F. Complications of external fixation of the wrist. *Injury* **1994**, *25* (Suppl. S4), S-d39-43. [CrossRef]
63. Burke, E.F.; Singer, R.M. Treatment of comminuted distal radius with the use of an internal distraction plate. *Tech. Hand Up. Extrem. Surg.* **1998**, *2*, 248–252. [CrossRef]
64. Dicpinigaitis, P.; Wolinsky, P.; Hiebert, R.; Egol, K.; Koval, K.; Tejwani, N. Can external fixation maintain reduction after distal radius fractures? *J. Trauma* **2004**, *57*, 845–850. [CrossRef] [PubMed]
65. Jorge-Mora, A.A.; Cecilia-López, D.; Rodríguez-Vega, V.; Suárez-Arias, L.; Andrés-Esteban, E.; Porras-Moreno, M.; Resines-Erasun, C. Comparison between external fixators and fixed-angle volar-locking plates in the treatment of distal radius fractures. *J. Hand Microsurg.* **2012**, *4*, 50–54. [CrossRef] [PubMed]

66. Richard, M.J.; Wartinbee, D.A.; Riboh, J.; Miller, M.; Leversedge, F.J.; Ruch, D.S. Analysis of the complications of palmar plating versus external fixation for fractures of the distal radius. *J. Hand Surg.* **2011**, *36*, 1614–1620. [CrossRef] [PubMed]
67. Williksen, J.H.; Frihagen, F.; Hellund, J.C.; Kvernmo, H.D.; Husby, T. Volar locking plates versus external fixation and adjuvant pin fixation in unstable distal radius fractures: A randomized, controlled study. *J. Hand Surg.* **2013**, *38*, 1469–1476. [CrossRef]
68. Maccagnano, G.; Noia, G.; Vicenti, G.; Coviello, M.; Pesce, V.; Moretti, B. A Prospective Observational Clinical and Radiological Study of a Modular Bridging External Fixator for Unstable Distal Radius Fractures. *Malays Orthop. J.* **2021**, *15*, 108–114. [CrossRef]
69. Mishra, R.K.; Sharma, B.P.; Kumar, A.; Sherawat, R. A comparative study of variable angle volar plate and bridging external fixator with K-wire augmentation in comminuted distal radius fractures. *Chin. J. Traumatol.* **2021**, *24*, 301–305. [CrossRef]
70. Aita, M.A.; Rodrigues, F.L.; Alves, K.; de Oliveira, R.K.; Ruggiero, G.M.; Rodrigues, L.M.R. Bridging versus Nonbridging Dynamic External Fixation of Unstable Distal Radius Fractures in the Elderly with Polytrauma: A Randomized Study. *J. Wrist Surg.* **2019**, *8*, 408–415. [CrossRef]
71. Ring, D.; Jupiter, J.B. Treatment of osteoporotic distal radius fractures. *Osteoporos. Int.* **2005**, *16*, S80–S84. [CrossRef]

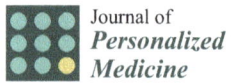

Article

The Impact of Hip Dysplasia on CAM Impingement

Carsten Y. W. Heimer [1], Chia H. Wu [2], Carsten Perka [1], Sebastian Hardt [1], Friedemann Göhler [3], Tobias Winkler [1,4,5,†] and Henrik C. Bäcker [1,*,†]

[1] Centrum für Muskuloskeletale Chirurgie, Charité—Universitätsmedizin Berlin, Augustenburger Platz 1, 13353 Berlin, Germany; carsten.heimer@charite.de (C.Y.W.H.); carsten.perka@charite.de (C.P.); sebastian.hardt@charite.de (S.H.); tobias.winkler@charite.de (T.W.)
[2] Department of Orthopaedics & Sports Medicine, Baylor College of Medicine Medical Centre, Houston, TX 77030, USA; wu.h.chia@gmail.com
[3] Department of Radiology, Charité Berlin, University Hospital, Charitéplatz 1, 10117 Berlin, Germany; friedemann.goehler@charite.de
[4] Julius Wolff Institute, Berlin Institute of Health at Charité—Universitätsmedizin Berlin, Augustenburger Platz 1, 13353 Berlin, Germany
[5] Berlin Institute of Health Center for Regenerative Therapies, Berlin Institute of Health at Charité—Universitätsmedizin Berlin, Augustenburger Platz 1, 13353 Berlin, Germany
* Correspondence: henrik.baecker@charite.de
† The authors contributed equally to this study.

Abstract: Predisposing factors for CAM-type femoroacetabular impingement (FAI) include acetabular protrusion and retroversion; however, nothing is known regarding development in dysplastic hips. The purpose of this study was to determine the correlation between CAM-type FAI and developmental dysplastic hips diagnosed using X-ray and rotational computed tomography. In this retrospective study, 52 symptomatic hips were included, with a mean age of 28.8 ± 7.6 years. The inclusion criteria consisted of consecutive patients who suffered from symptomatic dysplastic or borderline dysplastic hips and underwent a clinical examination, conventional radiographs and rotational computed tomography. Demographics, standard measurements and the rotational alignments were recorded and analyzed between the CAM and nonCAM groups. Among the 52 patients, 19 presented with CAM impingement, whereas, in 33 patients, no signs of CAM impingement were noticed. For demographics, no significant differences between the two groups were identified. On conventional radiography, the acetabular hip index as well as the CE angle for the development of CAM impingement were significantly different compared to the nonCAM group with a CE angle of 21.0° ± 5.4° vs. 23.7° ± 5.8° ($p = 0.050$) and an acetabular hip index of 25.6 ± 5.7 vs. 21.9 ± 7.3 ($p = 0.031$), respectively. Furthermore, a crossing over sign was observed to be more common in the nonCAM group, which is contradictory to the current literature. For rotational alignment, no significant differences were observed. In dysplastic hips, the CAM-type FAI correlated to a lower CE angle and a higher acetabular hip index. In contrast to the current literature, no significant correlations to the torsional alignment or to crossing over signs were observed.

Keywords: radiography; CAM; femoroacetabular; impingement; FAI; PAO; dysplasia; borderline

1. Introduction

The femoroacetabular impingement (FAI) pathology is not only correlated with hip pain but also predisposing for early onset osteoarthritis [1]. It results from an aspherical head–femoral neck junction (CAM type, Figure 1), which is often referred to as pistol grip or post-slip deformity, which typically causes shear stress at the labrum, and cartilage is typically in the anterosuperior region of the acetabulum (pincer type) [2]. These stresses are thought to separate labrum and cartilage, leading to articular degeneration and osteoarthritis [3,4]. Typical causes include acetabular protrusion or acetabular retroversion with anterior overcoverage of the femoral head [1,5]. Thus, especially acetabular retroversion correlated with the development of extra-articular subspace impingement, however, the location of impingement may differ. In addition to underlying biomechanical pathologies of the hip, the range of motion is thought to be important for the development of FAI, also causing an increased shear stress on the labrum and, subsequently, the cartilage [1].

In contrast to CAM-type impingement, the pincer type is not related to an asphericity of the femoral head. Typically, the cause is a deep socket, which limits the hip's range of motions related to an overcovering acetabular rim. Thus, the femoral neck abuts against the labrum, which is compressed. The forces are transmitted to the acetabular cartilage causing ossification [4].

The opposite of a larger femoral head coverage, such as protrusio acetabula, is developmental dysplasia of the hip (DDH). Typically, it is screened in infants to initiate treatment as early as possible and to allow for a good development of the acetabulum to avoid early onset of secondary hip osteoarthritis [6]. In adults, for diagnosis of DDH, a conventional radiography is performed, showing a low center edge angle, acetabular hip index and acetabular hip angle (AIA). Currently, little is known about the correlating rotational alignment [7] or the presence of CAM FAI in such cases. As a result, surgeons indicate periacetabular osteotomy in DDH without considering or approaching CAM FAIs. Even worse, if the acetabulum is repositioned, a larger femoral coverage can be achieved, which may worsen the development of CAM FAI and, therefore, secondary osteoarthritis.

Because of the dearth in the literature, this study aimed to investigate the radiographic correlation and underlying cause between CAM-type FAI and dysplastic respectively borderline dysplastic hips including the standard measurements of the hip and the rotational alignment of the lower extremity.

2. Materials and Methods

A retrospective chart review was performed between 2017 and 2019 after obtaining ethical approval (EA4/201/19). In the period of interest, all consecutive patients aged of 18 years or older presenting with dysplastic (type 2) and/or borderline dysplastic hips (type 1), both types defined by the CE angle, the sharp angle, the acetabular index angle or the presence of a crossing over sign, who underwent a rotational CT scan and two conventional radiographies were included. Further, demographics including age, gender, body weight, body height, body mass index (BMI) and comorbidities were noted. The exclusion criteria consisted of patients without pathological radiographical values, incomplete medical or radiographic charts, no accessible CT images and patients younger than 18 years of age.

The X-rays were performed anteroposteriorly for the pelvis as well as in an axial view and faux profile of the affected hip. In addition to the presence of a CAM femoroacetabular impingement, defined as an extra bone formation at the anterolateral head–neck junction leading to a non-spherical morphology of the femoral head, we analyzed standard measurements including center edge angle (CE), acetabular index angle (AI angle), sharp angle, hip lateralization index, acetabular hip index (AHI) and centrum-collum-diaphyseal angle (CCD) from an anteroposterior view as well as the alpha—vertical line parallel to either the outer and inner cortex of the ilium and the acetabular rim—and beta angles—vertical line parallel to either the outer or inner cortex of the ilium and the lowest and lateral most point of the bright spot of the lower limb of the os ilium—from an axial view. Furthermore, we recorded the presence of pincer-type impingement.

For rotational CT, nonenhanced CTs of the lower limb were obtained either on a 320-row or an 80-row CT scanner (Canon Aquilion ONE Vision Edition and Canon Aquilion PRIME, respectively, both Canon Medical Systems, Tochigi, Japan). Thus, a scanogram and a helical acquisition of the lower limb were obtained, and the scan was performed with 120 KVp tube voltage. An automated tube current modulation was set to the low-dose mode (standard deviation of 25). For image processing, iterative reconstruction (adaptive iterative dose reduction (AIDR) 3D standard) and a bone kernel (filter convolution (FC) 08-H) was used with CT images of 0.5 to 1.0 mm in thick slices.

Measurements were performed on the axial views of the lower limb scan and included the acetabular rotation, defined as the angle between the level of the tangent along the posterior and the anterior acetabular edge and a tangent along the right and left sciatic spina. Additionally, femoral torsion, tibial torsion and tibiofemoral torsion were calculated based on the measurements of the femoral neck (angle between a line through femoral neck and femoral head center and image base line), femoral condyle (angle between tangent along the posterior condyle border and image base line), tibial plateau (angle between a tangent along the posterior edge of the tibial plateau and image base line) and upper ankle rotation (angle between a line through the talus and the lateral malleolus and the image base line). Finally, the tibiofemoral rotation was calculated as the difference between the rotation of the femoral condyles and the rotation of the tibial plateau. All measurements were performed by a musculoskeletal trained radiologist.

The severity of DDH was classified into dysplastic and borderline dysplastic hips as published by Tannast et al. [8–11]. Therefore, a borderline dysplastic hip was defined as a CE angle between 20° and 24.9°, a sharp angle between 39 and 42° or combined acetabular retroversion (presence of a crossing over sign) with normal values. A dysplastic hip was defined as a CE angle less than 20°, an AI angle greater than 10°, a sharp angle greater than 42° or an AHI greater than 25° [8,9]. The physiological values for acetabular as well as femoral torsions were defined to be between 10° and 25° [12,13]. Two examples are shown in Figures 1 and 2.

A functional clinical examination was performed when the patients first presented in clinics. Thus, the range of motion, including flexion/extension, internal/external rotation and abduction/adduction, were assessed.

For statistical analysis, we used the IBM SPSS Statistics 26 Core System (IBM, Armonk, NY, USA). An ANOVA t-test and a mixed model were applied, because they encounter the dependent variable of the person. Additionally, a linear regression analysis was performed to identify cross-correlation significances. Normally distributed continuous variables are presented with the mean and standard deviation of the mean (SD). The level of significances was set to a (*) p-value ≤ 0.05.

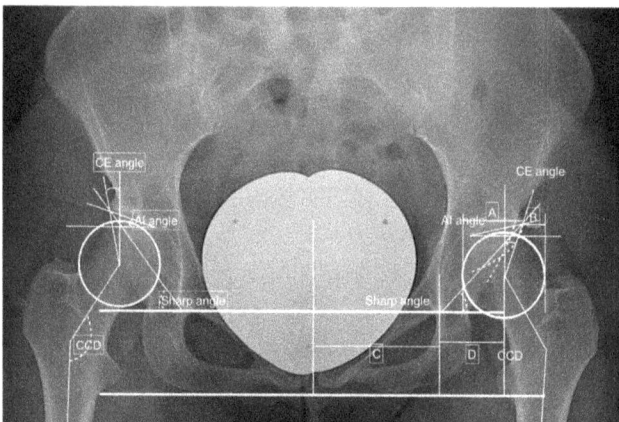

Figure 1. Preoperative findings and measurements performed. Left side: CE angle—between the Perkin line and the line between the center of the femoral head to the lateral edge of the acetabulum $-18.8°$; AI angle—between the Hilgenreiner's line and a parallel line to the acetabular roof—12.3°; sharp angle—between the horizontal teardrop line and a line connecting the teardrop to the lateral acetabulum—43.9°; hip lateralization index—quotient between the horizontal distance of the lateral femoral head that is uncovered by the acetabulum divided by a horizontal width of the femoral head—0.54; anterior hip index—quotient of the femoral head that is covered by the acetabular roof and the width of the femoral head—73.9; CCD angle—between the axis of the femoral diaphysis and the axis of the femoral neck—137.4° and positive crossing over sign. Adopted from [14,15].

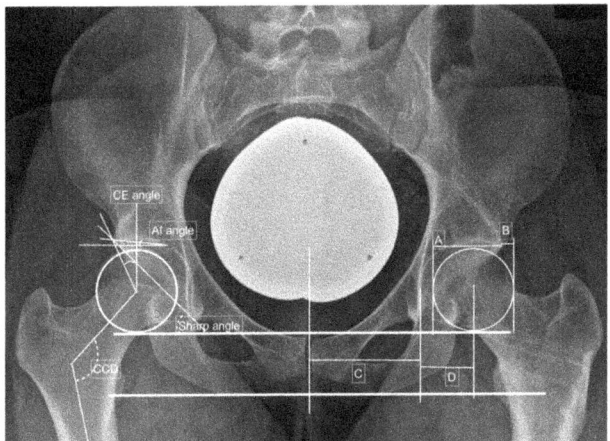

Figure 2. Preoperative measurements in a right-sided borderline dysplastic hip: CE angle—23.4°; AIA—4.9°; sharp angle—40.0°; hip lateralization—0.51; anterior hip index—82.8; CCD angle—121.0°. Adopted from [14,15].

3. Results

A total of 52 symptomatic hips of patients at a mean age of 28.8 ± 7.6 years were included. In nineteen of the patients, pathoanatomical parameters of a CAM impingement were observed, whereas in 33 patients, no CAM impingement was noticed. Female patients were predominant, representing 88.5% of cases (n = 46/52). The average height, body weight and body mass index (BMI) were 169.7 ± 8.4 cm, 68.1 ± 12.2 kg and 23.8 ± 4.3 kg/m². No significant differences between the two groups were identified as illustrated in Table 1.

Table 1. Demographics of the individuals presenting with symptomatic hip pain.

	Total	Coefficient	*p*-Value	CAM	nonCAM	*p*-Value
Numbers	52			19 (36.5%)	33 (63.5%)	
Female (%)	46 (88.5)	−0.139	0.520	16 (84.2)	30 (90.9)	0.238
Left hip (%)	25 (48.1)	−0.078	0.573	8 (42.1)	17 (51.5)	0.261
Age (years)	28.8 ± 7.6	0.014	0.134	30.9 ± 6.6	27.6 ± 7.9	0.067
Height (cm)	169.7 ± 8.4	0.013	0.822	171.6 ± 9.1	168.6 ± 7.9	0.125
Bodyweight (kg)	68.1 ± 12.2	−0.008	0.920	66.1 ± 9.7	69.4 ± 13.5	0.189
BMI (kg/m²)	23.8 ± 4.3	−0.003	0.990	22.4 ± 2.6	24.5 ± 5.0	0.059
Borderline DDH	13 (25.0%)	0.179	0.253	3 (15.8%)	10 (30.3%)	
DDH	39 (75.0%)	0.179	0.253	16 (84.2%)	23 (69.7%)	

In the functional clinical examination, no significant differences between the groups were observed for internal/external rotation, flexion/extension and abduction/adduction. All findings are presented in Table 2.

Table 2. Hip range of motion in the CAM and nonCAM groups.

	Coefficient	*p*-Value	Total	CAM	nonCAM	*p*-Value
Flexion (°)	−0.011	0.120	130 ± 13.1	132.6 ± 12.8	128.5 ± 13.4	0.139
Extension (°)	−0.026	0.111	2.1 ± 4.1	2.6 ± 4.5	1.8 ± 3.9	0.249
External rotation (°)	0.009	0.202	52.8 ± 11.5	54.5 ± 11.4	51.8 ± 11.6	0.214
Internal rotation (°)	0.006	0.280	41.4 ± 14.3	41.3 ± 14.8	41.4 ± 14.2	0.495
Abduction (°)	0.010	0.139	51.8 ± 15.2	51.8 ± 15.9	51.8 ± 15.1	0.498
Adduction (°)	−0.007	0.467	26.9 ± 10.0	29.0 ± 11.5	25.8 ± 9.0	0.136

For conventional radiography, significant differences between the CAM and nonCAM group were found for the CE angle as well as the acetabular hip index at 21.0 ± 5.4 vs. 23.7 ± 5.8 ($p = 0.050$) and 25.6 ± 5.7 vs. 21.9 ± 7.3 ($p = 0.031$), respectively. Further, a crossing over sign was identified to be more common in the nonCAM group ($p = 0.091$). In all cases, no pincer impingement was observed (Table 3).

Table 3. Findings on the anteroposterior pelvis radiographs and axial views of the affected hips.

	Total	Coefficient	p-Value	CAM	nonCAM	p-Value
CE angle (°)	22.7 ± 5.8	0.002	0.968	21.0 ± 5.4	23.7 ± 5.8	0.050
AI angle (°)	11.2 ± 5.2	0.006	0.781	12.6 ± 6.3	10.3 ± 4.3	0.065
Sharp angle (°)	42.5 ± 3.7	−0.005	0.894	43.3 ± 3.5	42.1 ± 3.8	0.148
Hip lateralization index	0.56 ± 0.06	0.617	0.590	0.57 ± 0.06	0.56 ± 0.06	0.214
AHI	23.2 ± 7.0	0.017	0.524	25.6 ± 5.7	21.9 ± 7.3	0.031
CCD (°)	133.0 ± 5.7	<0.005	0.994	133.3 ± 6.4	132.8 ± 5.4	0.378
Crossing over sign	17 (32.7)	−0.194	0.184	4 (21.1)	13 (39.4)	0.091
Kellgren–Lawrence score	0.4 ± 0.5	0.015	0.909	0.4 ± 0.5	0.4 ± 0.5	0.488
Alpha angle (°)	100.0 ± 10.9	−0.001	0.922	101.5 ± 10.0	98.8 ± 11.6	0.235
Beta angle (°)	57.0 ± 7.5	0.015	0.288	58.8 ± 7.8	55.7 ± 7.2	0.111

For the rotational alignment, no significant differences were observed between groups; however, positive tendencies were found for the tibial plateau torsion with −4.9 ± 9.4 (CAM) vs. −9.0° ± 10.7° (nonCAM) ($p = 0.084$). All findings for the torsional alignments are presented in Table 4.

Table 4. Rotational computed tomography findings.

	Total	Coefficient	p-Value	CAM	nonCAM	p-Value
Acetabular torsion (°)	18.9 ± 5.7	−0.005	0.712	18.6 ± 6.5	19.1 ± 5.3	0.373
Femoral neck torsion (°)	15.4 ± 10.7	0.012	0.516	15.7 ± 8.3	15.2 ± 12.0	0.432
Femoral condyle torsion (°)	−13.2 ± 9.8	−0.048	0.277	−12.4 ± 10.7	−13.7 ± 9.4	0.328
Femoral torsion (°)	27.7 ± 12.6	−0.014	0.469	26.5 ± 12.6	28.4 ± 12.7	0.305
Tibial plateau torsion (°)	−7.5 ± 10.4	0.042	0.305	−4.9 ± 9.4	−9.0 ± 10.7	0.084
Femorotibial torsion (°)	6.3 ± 5.0	−0.025	0.589	7.6 ± 6.5	5.5 ± 3.7	0.066
Ankle torsion (°)	28.9 ± 10.5	0.008	0.202	30.2 ± 11.2	27.9 ± 10.1	0.236
Tibial torsion (°)	37.0 ± 7.8	−0.008	0.336	36.6 ± 9.6	37.3 ± 6.5	0.377
Leg torsion (°)	−13.5 ± 14.0	−0.002	0.674	−14.5 ± 14.3	−12.8 ± 14.0	0.337

4. Discussion

Our results show that the pathology of CAM impingement in dysplastic and borderline dysplastic hips correlated significantly with the CE angle as well as the acetabular hip index. Positive tendencies were found for age and a lower BMI. On the other side, the rotational alignment of the lower extremity, especially of the femur and the acetabulum, did not affect the presence of CAM impingement in our cohort.

Although all patients who were included in this study presented with hip pain related to hip dysplasia, a combined FAI may exacerbate the symptoms. For definite radiographic diagnosis of FAI and DDH, a standardized X-ray, including an anteroposterior X-ray of the pelvis, an axial view and faux profile of the affected hip, is essential [16–19]. For diagnosis of intraarticular lesions, such as potential labral tears or chondral lesions, additional diagnostic tools, including rotational CT and MRI, are essential [20].

The current literature suggests that CAM impingement is found especially in young patients and typically associated with a countercoup lesion at the posterior inferior acetabular margin [21]. Biomechanically, larger total and anterior femoral head coverage in protrusio acetabula as well as acetabular retroversion or an extra-articular anterior supine hip impingement are described to be predisposing factors. Other correlating pathologies described in the literature include reduced femoral torsion [22] as well as an anterior iliac inferior spine [22,23]. For torsional alignment, a femoral retroversion (<5°) and increased femoral torsion (>35°) has been described to be associated with CAM impingement [24]. Another high prevalence described includes a combined femoral and tibial torsional abnormality with a mean femoral antetorsion of 23° and tibial antetorsion of 29° [25,26]. All these findings are thought to cause a mismatch between femoral head and acetabulum, leading to cartilage damage and, subsequently, to excessive growth of bone, the so-called os-acetabuli stress reaction, which can be identified as an asymmetry of the femoral head–neck junction [20]. For range of motion, limitations could be observed especially in hip flexion and internal rotation in the patients suffering from protrusio acetabula [1], whereas decreased femoral torsion showed less flexion and internal rotation in 90° flexion [22].

Wells J. et al. [27] investigated the proximal femoral characteristics and observed an incidence of cam deformity in 42%, which is comparable to the 36.5% in our cohort. Thus, the authors defined CAM-type FAI as an alpha angle greater than or equal to 55°; however, only 76% of patients tested positive for anterior impingement compared to 83% of patients with an alpha angle less than or equal to 55°. In the CAM-type FAI group, a reduced head–neck offset at the 1:30 point in 82% was noted, and a significant difference between mild and moderate-to-severe DDH was observed for femoral head–neck offset, respectively, with a femoral head–neck offset ratio of 12:00 (p = 0.04 and p = 0.01, respectively). For the femoral version in DDH, no significant correlation to the CAM-type FAI was observed [26]. In comparison to our trial, this study focused on the femoral characteristics and not the acetabular ones, except for the CE angle. Furthermore, no other torsional measurements were performed including acetabular torsion.

In our cohort, the acetabular hip index as well as CE were associated significantly with the development of CAM impingement. Thus, a low CE angle of 21.0° ± 5.4° (CAM) vs. 23.7° ± 5.8° (nonCAM) was significantly predisposing for impingement pathomorphology with a p-value of 0.05. For the acetabular hip index, a higher index of 25.6 ± 5.7 (CAM) compared to 21.9 ± 7.3 in the nonCAM group were observed (p = 0.031). This may be related to increased range of motion, especially of the abduction, causing chondral lesion at the head–neck junction. Another possible explanation could be the incomplete development of the hip in DDH, where the capsule is located more medial at the head–neck junction than in nonCAM hips. Subsequently, the acetabular hip index was higher avoiding any potential hip dislocation. Interestingly, a crossing over sign was identified to be more common in the nonCAM group, which is contradictory to the current literature. In DDH, a combination of retroversion may prevent too much range of motion and, therefore, prevent the development of CAM impingement. For femoral torsion, no significant differences were observed, although this was, overall, a bit higher than normal at 27.7° ± 12.6°. Likewise, with the torsional alignment, no correlation to the range of motion could be identified between the two groups.

For treatment, current guidelines for FAI suggest a symptomatic approach including acetabular trimming with hip arthroscopy, anterior inferior iliac spinal decompression and periacetabular osteotomies. The latter ones were discussed for reorientation, especially in retroverted hips with questionable outcome in the development of osteoarthritis [1], raising the question regarding which intrinsic factors may be involved in the development. These could either include genetic or epigenetic causes, such as collagen alpha-1(I) chain gene (COL1A1) and vitamin D receptor (VDR) [28,29], or an incomplete/inadequate chondrogenesis in DDH.

There were several limitations to this study. This study was of a retrospective design and only included 52 consecutive hips that were diagnosed with dysplastic and/or borderline dysplastic hips undergoing a rotational CT scan. Furthermore, to identify significant differences (p < 0.05) in the measurements between the CAM and nonCAM groups on the radiographs, small variations related to the positioning of the patient and the technique used to perform the X-rays could be observed. No long-term follow up was performed, which makes it difficult to discuss the development of osteoarthritis. Additionally, it was difficult to differentiate between the clinical symptoms resulting from the DDH abnormality or the FAI. Additionally, although no differences between DDH and borderline DDH were found, the subgroups were potentially underpowered. To minimize this error, all measurements of the plain radiography were performed by an orthopedic-surgeon trained observer and all measurements of the computed tomography by a specialized musculoskeletal trained radiologist. A consensus reading was not performed since the interobserver and intraobserver reliability were described as 0.911 and 0.955 for EOS, respectively, 0.934 and 0.934 for CT scan to measure the rotational alignment [30].

5. Conclusions

In dysplastic and borderline dysplastic hips, the AHI as well as the CE angle were significantly associated with the development of CAM impingement in our cohort. The crossing over sign was identified to be more common in the nonCAM group, which is contradictory to the current literature. These findings may suggest that in addition to the biomechanical abnormalities, intrinsic factors, including genetic and epigenetic causes, or incomplete chondrogenesis have an important role in the development of the FAI.

Author Contributions: All authors contributed to the study's conception and design. Material preparation, data collection and analyses were performed by C.Y.W.H., H.C.B. and F.G. The first draft of the manuscript was written by C.Y.W.H., H.C.B., C.H.W. and T.W. All authors commented on previous versions of the manuscript: C.Y.W.H., C.H.W., F.G., C.P., S.H., T.W. and H.C.B. All authors have read and agreed to the published version of the manuscript.

Funding: This research received no external funding.

Institutional Review Board Statement: The study was conducted in accordance with the Declaration of Helsinki and approved by the Institutional Review Board of the Charite Berlin, Germany (protocol code: EA4_201_19 and 12/11/2019).

Informed Consent Statement: Patient consent was waived due to the retrospective design.

Data Availability Statement: Not applicable.

Acknowledgments: We acknowledge support from the German Research Foundation (DFG) and the Open Access Publication Funds of Charité—Universitätsmedizin Berlin.

Conflicts of Interest: The authors declare no conflict of interest.

References

1. Lerch, T.D.; Siegfried, M.; Schmaranzer, F.; Leibold, C.S.; Zurmühle, C.A.; Hanke, M.S.; Ryan, M.K.; Steppacher, S.D.; Siebenrock, K.A.; Tannast, M. Location of Intra- and Extra-articular Hip Impingement Is Different in Patients with Pincer-Type and Mixed-Type Femoroacetabular Impingement Due to Acetabular Retroversion or Protrusio Acetabuli on 3D CT-Based Impingement Simulation. *Am. J. Sports Med.* **2020**, *48*, 661–672. [CrossRef] [PubMed]
2. Harris-Hayes, M.; Royer, N.K. Relationship of acetabular dysplasia and femoroacetabular impingement to hip osteoarthritis: A focused review. *PMR* **2011**, *3*, 1055–1067.e1. [CrossRef] [PubMed]
3. Ganz, R.; Parvizi, J.; Beck, M.; Leunig, M.; Nötzli, H.; Siebenrock, K. Femoroacetabular impingement: A cause for osteoarthritis of the hip. *Clin. Orthop. Relat. Res.* **2003**, *417*, 112–120.
4. Beck, M.; Kalhor, M.; Leunig, M.; Ganz, R. Hip morphology influences the pattern of damage to the acetabular cartilage: Femoroacetabular impingement as a cause of early osteoarthritis of the hip. *J. Bone Jt. Surg.-Br. Vol.* **2005**, *87*, 1012–1018. [CrossRef] [PubMed]
5. Reynolds, D.; Lucas, J.; Klaue, K. Retroversion of the acetabulum. A cause of hip pain. *J. Bone Jt. Surg.-Br. Vol.* **1999**, *81*, 281–288. [CrossRef]
6. Partenheimer, A.; Scheler-Hofmann, M.; Lange, J.; Kühl, R.; Follak, N.; Ebner, A.; Fusch, C.; Stenger, R.; Merk, H.; Haas, J.P. Correlation between sex, intrauterine position and familial predisposition and neonatal hip ultrasound results. *Ultraschall Med.* **2006**, *27*, 364–367. [CrossRef]
7. Beltran, L.S.; Rosenberg, Z.S.; Mayo, J.D.; De Tuesta, M.D.; Martin, O.; Neto, L.P.; Bencardino, J.T. Imaging evaluation of developmental hip dysplasia in the young adult. *AJR Am. J. Roentgenol.* **2013**, *200*, 1077–1088. [CrossRef]
8. Mannava, S.; Geeslin, A.G.; Frangiamore, S.J.; Cinque, M.E.; Geeslin, M.G.; Chahla, J.; Philippon, M.J. Comprehensive Clinical Evaluation of Femoroacetabular Impingement: Part 2, Plain Radiography. *Arthrosc. Tech.* **2017**, *6*, e2003–e2009. [CrossRef]
9. Henle, P.; Tannast, M.; Siebenrock, K.A. Imaging in developmental dysplasia of the hip. *Orthopade* **2008**, *37*, 525–531. [CrossRef]
10. Sharp, I.K. Acetabular Dysplasia—The Acetabular Angle. *J. Bone Jt. Surg.-Br. Vol.* **1961**, *43*, 268–272. [CrossRef]

11. Tannast, M.; Hanke, M.S.; Zheng, G.; Steppacher, S.D.; Siebenrock, K.A. What are the radiographic reference values for acetabular under- and overcoverage? *Clin. Orthop. Relat. Res.* **2015**, *473*, 1234–1246. [CrossRef] [PubMed]
12. Tonnis, D.; Heinecke, A. Acetabular and femoral anteversion: Relationship with osteoarthritis of the hip. *J Bone Jt. Surg Am.* **1999**, *81*, 1747–1770. [CrossRef] [PubMed]
13. Waidelich, H.A.; Strecker, W.; Schneider, E. Computed tomographic torsion-angle and length measurement of the lower extremity. The methods, normal values and radiation load. *Rofo* **1992**, *157*, 245–251. [CrossRef]
14. Tannast, M.; Siebenrock, K.A.; Anderson, S.E. Femoroacetabular impingement: Radiographic diagnosis–what the radiologist should know. *AJR Am. J. Roentgenol.* **2007**, *188*, 1540–1552. [CrossRef] [PubMed]
15. Heimer, C.Y.W.; Göhler, F.; Vosseller, J.T.; Hardt, S.; Perka, C.; Bäcker, H.C. Rotation abnormalities in dysplastic hips and how to predict acetabular torsion. *Eur Radiol.* **2022**, 1–14.
16. Heimer, C.Y.W.; Wu, C.H.; Perka, C.; Hardt, S.; Göhler, F.; Bäcker, H.C. The impact of the Laterality on Radiographic Outcomes of the Bernese Periacetabular Osteotomy. *J. Pers. Med.* **2022**, *12*, 1072. [CrossRef]
17. Zheng, G.; Tannast, M.; Anderegg, C.; Siebenrock, K.A.; Langlotz, F. Hip2Norm: An object-oriented cross-platform program for 3D analysis of hip joint morphology using 2D pelvic radiographs. *Comput. Methods Programs Biomed.* **2007**, *87*, 36–45. [CrossRef]
18. Tannast, M.; Mistry, S.; Steppacher, S.D.; Reichenbach, S.; Langlotz, F.; Siebenrock, K.A.; Zheng, G. Radiographic analysis of femoroacetabular impingement with Hip2Norm-reliable and validated. *J. Orthop. Res.* **2008**, *26*, 1199–1205. [CrossRef]
19. Tannast, M.; Kubiak-Langer, M.; Langlotz, F.; Puls, M.; Murphy, S.B.; Siebenrock, K.A. Noninvasive three-dimensional assessment of femoroacetabular impingement. *J. Orthop. Res.* **2007**, *25*, 122–131. [CrossRef]
20. Anderson, S.E.; Siebenrock, K.A.; Tannast, M. Femoroacetabular impingement. *Eur. J. Radiol.* **2012**, *81*, 3740–3744. [CrossRef]
21. Pfirrmann, C.W.; Mengiardi, B.; Dora, C.; Kalberer, F.; Zanetti, M.; Hodler, J. Cam and pincer femoroacetabular impingement: Characteristic MR arthrographic findings in 50 patients. *Radiology* **2006**, *240*, 778–785. [CrossRef] [PubMed]
22. Lerch, T.D.; Boschung, A.; Todorski, I.A.; Steppacher, S.D.; Schmaranzer, F.; Zheng, G.; Ryan, M.K.; Siebenrock, K.A.; Tannast, M. Femoroacetabular Impingement Patients With Decreased Femoral Version Have Different Impingement Locations and Intra- and Extraarticular Anterior Subspine FAI on 3D-CT-Based Impingement Simulation: Implications for Hip Arthroscopy. *Am. J. Sports Med.* **2019**, *47*, 3120–3132. [CrossRef] [PubMed]
23. Hetsroni, I.; Poultsides, L.; Bedi, A.; Larson, C.M.; Kelly, B.T. Anterior inferior iliac spine morphology correlates with hip range of motion: A classification system and dynamic model. *Clin. Orthop. Relat. Res.* **2013**, *471*, 2497–2503. [CrossRef] [PubMed]
24. Lerch, T.D.; Schmaranzer, F.; Hanke, M.S.; Leibold, C.; Steppacher, S.D.; Siebenrock, K.A.; Tannast, M. Torsional deformities of the femur in patients with femoroacetabular impingement: Dynamic 3D impingement simulation can be helpful for the planning of surgical hip dislocation and hip arthroscopy. *Orthopade* **2020**, *49*, 471–481. [CrossRef]
25. Lerch, T.D.; Liechti, E.F.; Todorski, I.A.S.; Schmaranzer, F.; Steppacher, S.D.; Siebenrock, K.A.; Tannast, M.; Klenke, F.M. Prevalence of combined abnormalities of tibial and femoral torsion in patients with symptomatic hip dysplasia and femoroacetabular impingement. *Bone Jt. J.* **2020**, *102-B*, 1636–1645. [CrossRef]
26. Georgiadis, A.G.; Siegal, D.S.; Scher, C.E.; Zaltz, I. Can femoral rotation be localized and quantified using standard CT measures? *Clin. Orthop. Relat. Res.* **2015**, *473*, 1309–1314. [CrossRef]
27. Wells, J.; Nepple, J.J.; Crook, K.; Ross, J.R.; Bedi, A.; Schoenecker, P.; Clohisy, J.C. Femoral Morphology in the Dysplastic Hip: Three-dimensional Characterizations With CT. *Clin. Orthop. Relat. Res.* **2017**, *475*, 1045–1054. [CrossRef]
28. Zamborsky, R.; Kokavec, M.; Harsanyi, S.; Attia, D.; Danisovic, L. Developmental Dysplasia of Hip: Perspectives in Genetic Screening. *Med. Sci.* **2019**, *7*, 59. [CrossRef]
29. Jawadi, A.H.; Wakeel, A.; Tamimi, W.; Nasr, A.; Iqbal, Z.; Mashhour, A.; Fattah, M.A.; Alkhanein, N.; Abu Jaffal, A.S. Association analysis between four vitamin D receptor gene polymorphisms and developmental dysplasia of the hip. *J. Genet.* **2018**, *97*, 925–930. [CrossRef]
30. Mayr, H.O.; Schmidt, J.-P.; Haasters, F.; Bernstein, A.; Schmal, H.; Prall, W.C. Anteversion Angle Measurement in Suspected Torsional Malalignment of the Femur in 3-Dimensional EOS vs Computed Tomography-A Validation Study. *J. Arthroplast.* **2021**, *36*, 379–386. [CrossRef]

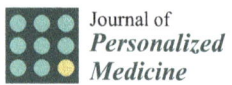

Article

Distal Radius Fracture with Ipsilateral Elbow Dislocation: A Rare but Challenging Injury

Henrik C. Bäcker [1,*,†], Kathi Thiele [1,†], Chia H. Wu [2], Philipp Moroder [1], Ulrich Stöckle [1] and Karl F. Braun [1,3]

1   Department of Orthopaedic Surgery and Traumatology, Charité Berlin, University Hospital Berlin, 10117 Berlin, Germany; kathi.thiele@charite.de (K.T.); philipp.moroder@charitee.de (P.M.); ulrich.stockle@charitee.de (U.S.); karl.braun@charitee.de (K.F.B.)
2   Department of Orthopaedics & Sports Medicine, Baylor College of Medicine Medical Centre, Houston, 77030 TX, USA; wu.chia.h@gmail.com
3   Department of Trauma Surgery, Technical University Munich, Klinikum Rechts der Isar, 81675 Munich, Germany
*   Correspondence: henrik.baecker@sports-med.org
†   The authors contributed equally to this study.

Abstract: Distal radius fractures are common and account for approximately 14% to 18% of all adult extremity injuries. On rare occasions, ipsilateral elbow dislocation can be observed additionally. However, this can be missed without careful examination, especially in patients experiencing altered mental status. The aim of this study was to analyze the mechanism, level of injury, demographics, and associated injuries in distal radius fracture with ipsilateral elbow dislocation. Between 2012 and 2019, we searched our trauma database for distal radius fracture with ipsilateral elbow dislocation. All patients older than 18 years old were included. Data on demographics, mechanism of injury, level of energy, and subsequent treatment were collected. A total of seven patients were identified. The mean age in this cohort was 68.7 ± 13.3 years old, and the left side was involved in 71.4% of the patients. Females were affected in 85.7% ($n = 6/7$) of cases, all of whom suffered from low-energy mono-trauma at a mean age of 71.5 ± 12.3 years old. One male patient suffered from high-energy trauma (52 years old). Mainly, posterior elbow dislocations were observed (66.7%; $n = 4/6$). Distal radius fracture patterns, in accordance with the AO classification, included two C2-, two C3-, one C1-, and one B1-type fractures. In the patient suffering from high-energy trauma, the closed distal radius fracture was classified as type C3. Associated injures included open elbow dislocation, ulnar artery rupture, and damage to the flexor digitorum superficialis. Although distal radius fracture with ipsilateral elbow dislocation is thought to be from high-energy trauma, this study shows that most patients were elderly females suffering from low-energy mechanisms. It is important for clinicians to maintain a high level of suspicion for any concomitant injury in this population.

Keywords: distal radius; elbow dislocation; treatment; epidemiology

Citation: Bäcker, H.C.; Thiele, K.; Wu, C.H.; Moroder, P.; Stöckle, U.; Braun, K.F. Distal Radius Fracture with Ipsilateral Elbow Dislocation: A Rare but Challenging Injury. *J. Pers. Med.* 2022, 12, 1097. https://doi.org/10.3390/jpm12071097

Academic Editor: Jih-Yang Ko

Received: 13 May 2022
Accepted: 29 June 2022
Published: 1 July 2022

Publisher's Note: MDPI stays neutral with regard to jurisdictional claims in published maps and institutional affiliations.

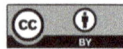

Copyright: © 2022 by the authors. Licensee MDPI, Basel, Switzerland. This article is an open access article distributed under the terms and conditions of the Creative Commons Attribution (CC BY) license (https://creativecommons.org/licenses/by/4.0/).

1. Introduction

Isolated distal radius fractures are one of the most common injuries and account for between 14% and 18% of all adult extremity injuries [1,2]. Risk factors include osteoporosis, White race, and female sex. Osteoporosis has been diagnosed in 64% of patients following screening [3]. Furthermore, most patients suffer from a fall in the winter months related to slippery walking conditions [4]. For treatment, a large variety of techniques have been described.

When looking for elbow instability, this is the second most common dislocated major joint after the shoulder [5,6]. It commonly occurs in young male patients with an odds ratio of 1.7–1.8:1 [7]. Most patients are under the age of 30 years [8,9], with peak incidence occurring between 5 and 25 years of age [5]. However, this pattern is different in the elderly population where more women are affected [10]. The dislocation is classified according to the direction of the ulna dislocation, of which posterior dislocation is the most common, seen in up to 79% of cases [11,12].

In patients who fall on outstretched arm, the loads are typically directed through either the distal radius alone or the elbow. Therefore, combined injuries are rare, and few case reports have been described [13,14]. For distal radius fractures, the wrist is typically in dorsiflexion, where the position of the wrist at the moment of impact determines the fracture pattern and concomitant injuries, if any. Pronation, supination, and abduction determine the direction of the force transmission [15]. Similarly, elbow dislocations typically occur from falling onto the extended arm [11] [16]. For posterior elbow dislocation, which is the most common dislocation type (>80% of cases), the injury mechanism is typically described as a combination of axial compression and valgus stress with the forearm supinated and elbow flexed [17–19]. For anterior elbow dislocation, the mechanism of injury is an anterior directed force on the proximal ulna with the elbow flexed in most cases [20].

The aim of this study was to investigate the epidemiology, demographics, diagnostic modalities, and subsequent treatment options for distal radius fractures with ipsilateral elbow dislocation at a major level 1 trauma center.

2. Materials and Methods

For this retrospective trial, we searched our trauma database between 2012 and 2019 for patients suffering from distal radius fracture with ipsilateral elbow dislocation. Patients older than 18 years of age presenting with a distal radius fracture and ipsilateral elbow dislocation in our emergency department were included. All patients suffering from any elbow fracture were excluded. Clinical records and radiographies were analyzed by a fellowship-trained orthopedic trauma surgeon. Data on age, gender, mechanism of injury, diagnostic modalities, neurologic deficits, fracture pattern of the distal radius, and any subsequent treatments rendered were recorded. Patients were classified according to the mechanism of injury including low (e.g., ground level fall) and high (e.g., motorcycle crash or fall from height). Furthermore, conventional radiographs and computed tomography images were analyzed for fracture patterns. Therefore, the AO/OTA classification was used to classify distal radius fractures. Elbow dislocations were classified according to the direction of dislocation. Information on any other concomitant injuries and comorbidities was noted.

For statistical analysis, Microsoft Excel (Microsoft Corporation, Redmond, WA, USA) and SPSS version 22 (IBM, Armonk, NY, USA) were used. For normally distributed values, the mean and standard error of the mean were calculated.

3. Results

In total, nine patients were found when searching our database between 2012 and 2020. There were two patients who suffered from elbow fractures and, as such, were excluded, leaving seven patients for final inclusion. The mean age was 68.7 ± 13.3 years old, ranging from 52 to 89 years old. Females consisted of 85.7% of cases ($n = 6/7$), and the left side was affected in 71.4% ($n = 5/7$) of cases (Table 1).

Table 1. Demographics of the patients suffering from distal radius fractures and ipsilateral elbow dislocation.

	Numbers (%)
Number of patients (n)	7 (100)
Gender (female)	6 (85.7)
Age (years)	65.3 ± 15.4
Level of energy (low energy)	6 (85.7)
Side (left)	5 (62.5)

Most patients in this study presented with low-energy trauma in 85.7% of cases (n = 6/7). In one patient, a high-energy mechanism was described, suffering from a fall from approximately 4 m in height (13 feet). Patients presenting with a low-energy mechanism suffered from monotrauma, whereas the one patient who sustained a high-energy mechanism sustained multiple injuries.

3.1. Low-Energy Injuries

The mean age of the patients with low-energy injuries was 71.5 ± 12.3 years old. Concerning distal radius fracture patterns, C types were observed in 83.3% of cases (n = 5/6), including two type C2, two type C3, one type C1, and one type B1. Furthermore, one patient suffered from an open distal radius fracture. Two patients sustained radiocarpal dislocation. No other concomitant injuries, such as neurovascular injuries, were observed. In all patients, elbow reduction was performed in the emergency room. Two patients underwent external fixation as initial treatment. In one case, external fixation was indicated for both elbow and wrist, and in another patient, it was only indicated for the wrist. For the remaining patients, the elbow was stable once reduced. Surgery was indicated in five patients consisting of a volar plate osteosynthesis, and in one patient addition suture anchors were required in order to stabilize the elbow. Conservative treatment was indicated in the nondisplaced B3-type distal radius fracture. This was treated with casting. In patients with stable elbow, the elbow was immobilized for one week, followed by a limited active range of motion in a hinged elbow brace allowing 20° to 90° of flexion for three weeks. Afterwards, patients were allowed a range of motion as tolerated without lifting of heavy weights for another two weeks. After operative treatment of the distal radius, active mobilization was allowed from day one while maintaining non-weight bearing. In all patients, a good to excellent range of motion (0°/0°/150°) of the elbow or wrist was achieved after intensive physiotherapy.

3.2. High-Energy Injuries

Only one male patient suffered from isolated distal radius fracture and elbow dislocation. At the time of accident, he was younger than the average age in the low-energy group. The left side was affected, and an open elbow dislocation was noted with an ulnar artery disruption. Other injuries included a pneumothorax on the left side, several rib fractures, spinopelvic dissociation type II, acetabulum fracture, and five lumbar transverse process fractures. Initially, damage control surgery was performed. This included temporary external fixation of the elbow and wrist, repair of the ulnar artery, local debridement, and application artificial skin substitute on the open wound. Once clinically stable, a combination of a volar plate and mini frag plate was used to fix the distal radius and distal ulnar fracture, respectively. For the elbow, lateral ulnar collateral ligament (LUCL) reconstruction was performed using two suture anchors. Postoperatively, the patient showed a limited range of motion in the elbow and the wrist. All injuries are illustrated in Table 2. In addition, one example is shown in Figure 1.

Table 2. Differentiation between low- and high-energy-related accidents, diagnoses, and subsequent treatments.

	Number (%)	Gender (Female)	Age (Years)	Distal Radius Fracture	Colles Fracture (%)	Elbow Dislocation	External Fixation	Volar Plate ORIF (%)	Elbow Stabilization (%)	Concomitant Injuries
Low-energy injuries	6 (85.7)	6 (100)	71.5 ± 12.3	1xB1; 1xC1; 2xC2; 2xC3	4 (57.1)	4 post.; 1 post-lat; 1 divergent	1 wrist; 1 elbow	5 (83.3)	1 (16.7)	1 – open fx
High-energy injuries	1 (14.3)	0 (0)	52	1xC3	1 (100)	unclear	1 elbow and wrist	1 (100)	1 (100)	1 – open fx and ulnar artery lesion
Total	7 (100)	6 (85.7)	65.3 ± 15.4					6	2 (28.6)	

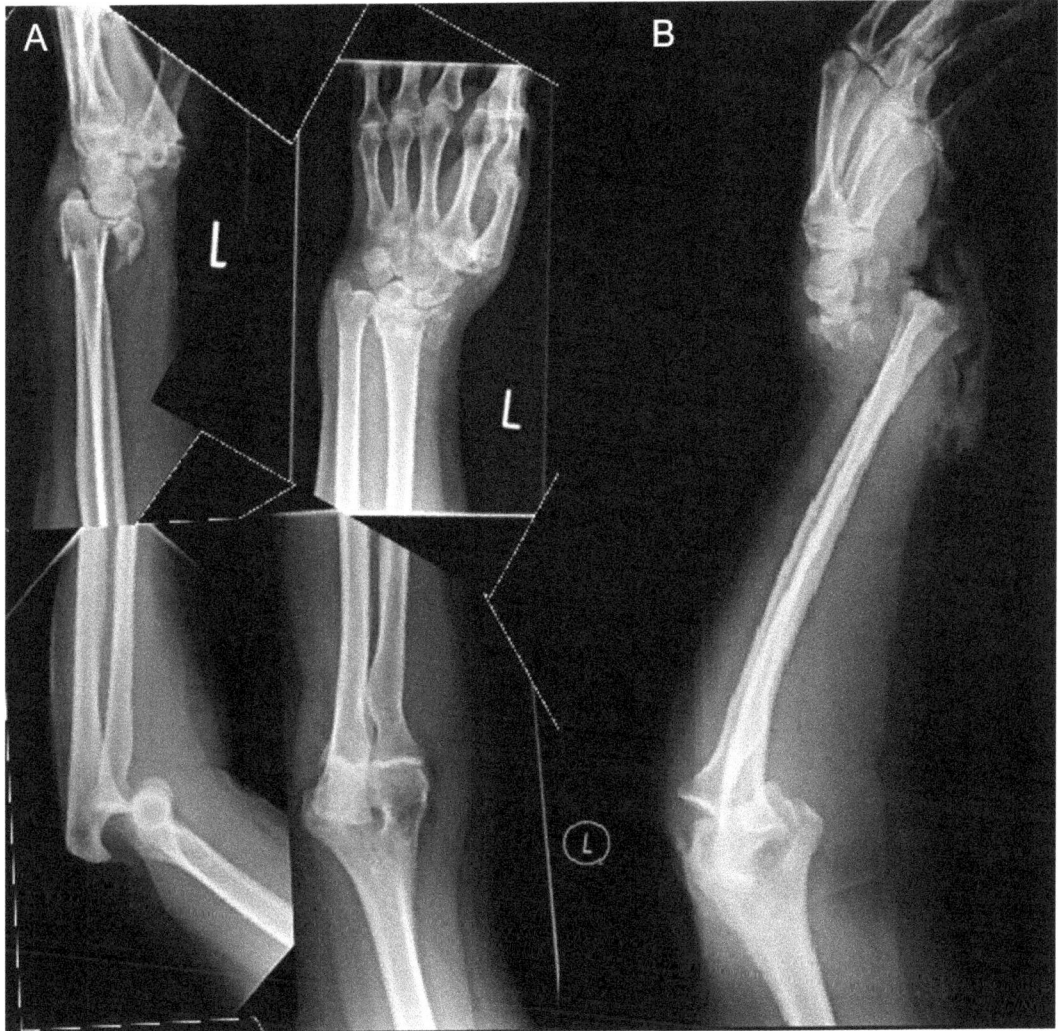

Figure 1. Female patients after low-energy falls with (**A**) a distal radius type-C3 fracture with posterior elbow dislocation and (**B**) an open distal radius type-C3 fracture with a concomitant posterolateral elbow dislocation.

4. Discussion

This study showed that combined distal radius fracture and ipsilateral elbow dislocation is most commonly sustained by elderly patients over the mean age of 70 years with a low-energy mechanism. In those with altered mental status, clinicians need to maintain a high degree of clinical suspicion to avoid missing concomitant injuries. Careful history and physical examination is imperative.

The existing literature tends to focus on isolated distal radius fractures or diaphyseal radial versus ulnar fractures with elbow dislocation [21,22]. There is relatively little published on distal radius fractures with ipsilateral elbow dislocation as it is uncommon. To our knowledge, our paper represents the largest cohort that has been published to date. The most commonly described injury mechanism includes axial loading on an outstretched hand with a supinated forearm and slightly flexed elbow [2]. The distal radius breaks initially due to the direct contact with the ground. Further, forces may transmit through the elbow, causing posteromedial dislocation [14]. Posteromedial dislocation is associated with axial loading of the elbow in a varus position and the forearm in pronation. Specific to our cohort, patients predominantly suffered from a directly posterior elbow dislocation.

While elbow dislocations are more frequently described in young male patients [7,9], most patients in our cohort were elderly females suffering from low-energy trauma. This may be due to the fact that we excluded any elbow fracture dislocation in our cohort. In a few cases, it is possible that a dislocation spontaneously reduced prior to presentation due to the fact of muscle contraction. It is also possible that the elbow unknowingly reduced when attempting closed reduction of the distal radius fracture. A thorough history and physical examination is crucial in patients where a concomitant injury is suspected.

While the use of plain film and computed tomography to assess fracture morphology is widely accepted, there is no consensus regarding the use of dynamic fluoroscopy as well as MRI to assess instability of the elbow joint. In particular, dynamic fluoroscopy allows detection of subtle instability throughout range of motion. MRI may allow assessment of the quality of soft tissue but does not allow assessment of how the tissue functions under stress. Surgical intervention is not routinely recommended for simple elbow dislocation. It is performed only if there is instability post-reduction, most commonly seen in extension.

Initially management of this combination of injuries typically involves closed reduction of the elbow and distal radius. Intravenous sedation is recommended to avoid patient duress and muscle relaxation while performing the reduction. Elbow stability should ideally be assessed under fluoroscopy in flexion and extension, valgus and varus, as well as pronation and supination [23]. In some cases, recurrent dislocation or subtle instability may be present in extension [16]. This is followed by closed reduction of the wrist, being mindful not to further traumatize the elbow. The elbow and wrist are then stabilized in a posterior long arm splint in 90 degrees of flexion.

In posterolateral elbow dislocations, the forearm should be pronated, whereas in posteromedial dislocations, it should be supinated when splinting. Subtle instability only present in extension can often be treated in a hinge elbow brace. This allows immobilization of the elbow in 90 degrees of flexion that can be advanced gradually to full extension. In the absence of instability post-reduction, early mobilization should be initiated to maintain functionality. This includes active assisted exercises starting in week 2 after injury. In patients where there is associated elbow fracture or gross instability, surgery is recommended to restore stability [24,25].

In our cohort, only two patients required surgical intervention: one suffered from an acute high-energy injury and one from a low-energy injury. For surgical stabilization, repair of the lateral ulnar collateral ligament (LUCL) was performed after several debridements of the elbow. In the second patient, repair of the capsule, medial, and lateral collateral ligaments were necessary to achieve stability. However, in the remaining five patients, conservative treatments were performed without any chronic instability.

5. Conclusions

Distal radius fracture with ipsilateral elbow dislocation without fracture is a rare type of injury. In our cohort, this most commonly affected elderly patients with a low-energy mechanism of injury. The most common type of dislocation was direct posterior, and most could be treated with closed reduction without surgical stabilization. Any subtle instability should be accessed via dynamic fluoroscopy. Surgical stabilization is recommended for gross instability. Physicians must be wary of any elbow pain in patients who present with distal radius fractures. A careful history, physical exam, and relevant imaging is imperative.

Author Contributions: Conceptualization, H.C.B. and K.T.; methodology, H.C.B. and K.T.; software, H.C.B.; validation, H.C.B., C.H.W., and K.F.B.; formal analysis, H.C.B.; investigation, H.C.B.; resources, U.S.; data curation, H.C.B.; writing—original draft preparation, H.C.B. and K.T.; writing—review and editing, H.C.B., K.T., K.F.B., P.M., U.S. and C.H.W.; visualization, H.C.B.; supervision, U.S.; project administration, H.C.B. All authors have read and agreed to the published version of the manuscript.

Funding: This research received no external funding.

Institutional Review Board Statement: The study was conducted in accordance with the Declaration of Helsinki and approved by the Institutional Review Board of Charité Berlin on 08.01.2022 (EA1/283/21).

Informed Consent Statement: Patient consent was waived due to the retrospective design by the ethical committee, Charite Berlin, EA1/283/21.

Data Availability Statement: All data are presented in the manuscript.

Acknowledgments: We acknowledge support from the German Research Foundation (DFG) and the Open Access Publication Funds of Charité-Universitätsmedizin Berlin.

Conflicts of Interest: The authors declare no conflict of interest.

References

1. Simic, P.M.; Weiland, A.J. Fractures of the distal aspect of the radius: Changes in treatment over the past two decades. *Instr. Course Lect.* **2003**, *52*, 185–195. [CrossRef] [PubMed]
2. AkmaKamaludin, N.A.; FerdausKamudin, N.A.; Abdullah, S.; Sapuan, J. Ipsilateral proximal and distal radius fractures with unstable elbow joint: Which should we address first? *Chin. J. Traumatol.* **2019**, *22*, 59–62. [CrossRef] [PubMed]
3. Sarfani, S.; Scrabeck, T.; Kearns, A.E.; Berger, R.A.; Kakar, S. Clinical efficacy of a fragility care program in distal radius fracture patients. *J. Hand Surg. Am.* **2014**, *39*, 664–669. [CrossRef] [PubMed]
4. Levin, L.S.; Rozell, J.C.; Pulos, N. Distal Radius Fractures in the Elderly. *J. Am. Acad. Orthop. Surg.* **2017**, *25*, 179–187. [CrossRef]
5. Stoneback, J.W.; Owens, B.D.; Sykes, J.; Athwal, G.S.; Pointer, L.; Wolf, J.M. Incidence of elbow dislocations in the United States population. *J. Bone Jt. Surg. Am.* **2012**, *94*, 240–245. [CrossRef]
6. Kuhn, M.A.; Ross, G. Acute elbow dislocations. *Orthop. Clin. N. Am.* **2008**, *39*, 155–161. [CrossRef]
7. Neviaser, J.S.; Wickstrom, J.K. Dislocation of the elbow: A retrospective study of 115 patients. *South Med. J.* **1977**, *70*, 172–173. [CrossRef]
8. Mehlhoff, T.L.; Noble, P.C.; Bennett, J.B.; Tullos, H.S. Simple dislocation of the elbow in the adult. Results after closed treatment. *J. Bone Jt. Surg. Am.* **1988**, *70*, 244–249. [CrossRef]
9. Josefsson, P.O.; Nilsson, B.E. Incidence of elbow dislocation. *Acta Orthop. Scand.* **1986**, *57*, 537–538. [CrossRef]
10. Robinson, P.M.; Griffiths, E.; Watts, A.C. Simple elbow dislocation. *Shoulder Elbow* **2017**, *9*, 195–204. [CrossRef]
11. Grazette, A.J.; Aquilina, A. The Assessment and Management of Simple Elbow Dislocations. *Open Orthop. J.* **2017**, *11*, 1373–1379. [CrossRef] [PubMed]
12. Muhlenfeld, N.; Frank, J.; Lustenberger, T.; Marzi, I.; Sander, A.L. Epidemiology and treatment of acute elbow dislocations: Current concept based on primary surgical ligament repair of unstable simple elbow dislocations. *Eur. J. Trauma Emerg. Surg.* **2020**, *48*, 629–636. [CrossRef] [PubMed]
13. Tiwari, V.; Karkhur, Y.; Das, A. Concomitant Posterolateral Elbow Dislocation with Ipsilateral Comminuted Intra-articular Distal Radius Fracture: A Rare Orthopaedic Scenario. *Cureus* **2018**, *10*, e2264. [CrossRef]
14. Meena, S.; Trikha, V.; Kumar, R.; Saini, P.; Sambharia, A.K. Elbow dislocation with ipsilateral distal radius fracture. *J. Nat. Sci. Biol. Med.* **2013**, *4*, 479–481. [CrossRef] [PubMed]
15. Havemann, D.; Busse, F.W. Accident mechanisms and classification in distal radius fracture. In *Langenbecks Archiv fur Chirurgie*; Supplement II; Verhandlungen der Deutschen Gesellschaft fur Chirurgie; Deutsche Gesellschaft fur Chirurgi: Berlin, Germany, 1990; pp. 639–642.
16. Layson, J.; Best, B.J. *Elbow Dislocation*; StatPearls: Treasure Island, FL, USA, 2020.
17. Taylor, F.; Sims, M.; Theis, J.C.; Herbison, G.P. Interventions for treating acute elbow dislocations in adults. *Cochrane Database Syst. Rev.* **2012**, *4*, CD007908. [CrossRef]
18. Biberthaler, P.; Kanz, K.G.; Siebenlist, S. Elbow joint dislocation—Important considerations for closed reduction. *MMW Fortschr. Der Med.* **2015**, *157*, 50–52.
19. O'Driscoll, S.W. How Do Elbows Dislocate?: Commentary on an article by Marc Schnetzke, MD; et al.: "Determination of Elbow Laxity in a Sequential Soft-Tissue Injury Model. A Cadaveric Study". *J. Bone Jt. Surg. Am.* **2018**, *100*, e46. [CrossRef]
20. Saouti, R.; Albassir, A.; Berger, J.P.; Fatemi, F.; Willems, S. Anterior elbow dislocation with recurrent instability. *Acta Orthop. Belg.* **2003**, *69*, 197–200.
21. Siebenlist, S.; Buchholz, A.; Braun, K.F. Fractures of the proximal ulna: Current concepts in surgical management. *EFORT Open Rev.* **2019**, *4*, 1–9. [CrossRef]
22. Hung, S.C.; Huang, C.K.; Chiang, C.C.; Chen, T.H.; Chen, W.M.; Lo, W.H. Monteggia type I equivalent lesion: Diaphyseal ulna and radius fractures with a posterior elbow dislocation in an adult. *Arch. Orthop. Trauma Surg.* **2003**, *123*, 311–313. [CrossRef]
23. Mathew, P.K.; Athwal, G.S.; King, G.J. Terrible triad injury of the elbow: Current concepts. *J. Am. Acad. Orthop. Surg.* **2009**, *17*, 137–151. [CrossRef] [PubMed]

24. Sandmann, G.H.; Siebenlist, S.; Lenich, A.; Neumaier, M.; Ahrens, P.; Kirchhoff, C.; Braun, K.F.; Lucke, M.; Biberthaler, P. Traumatic elbow dislocations in bouldering. *Unfallchirurg* **2014**, *117*, 274–280. [CrossRef] [PubMed]
25. Cohen, M.S.; Hastings, H., II. Acute elbow dislocation: Evaluation and management. *J. Am. Acad. Orthop. Surg.* **1998**, *6*, 15–23. [CrossRef] [PubMed]

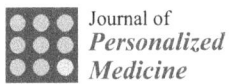

Article

The Impact of the Laterality on Radiographic Outcomes of the Bernese Periacetabular Osteotomy

Carsten Y. W. Heimer [1,*], Chia H. Wu [2], Carsten Perka [1], Sebastian Hardt [1], Friedemann Göhler [3] and Henrik C. Bäcker [1]

1 Department of Orthopaedic Surgery and Traumatology, Charité Berlin University Hospital, 10117 Berlin, Germany; carsten.perka@charite.de (C.P.); sebastian.hardt@charite.de (S.H.); henrik.baecker@sports-med.org (H.C.B.)
2 Department of Orthopaedics & Sports Medicine, Baylor College of Medicine Medical Centre, Houston, TX 77030, USA; wu.chia.h@gmail.com
3 Department of Radiology, Charité Berlin University Hospital, 10117 Berlin, Germany; friedemann.goehler@charite.de
* Correspondence: carsten.heimer@charite.de

Citation: Heimer, C.Y.W.; Wu, C.H.; Perka, C.; Hardt, S.; Göhler, F.; Bäcker, H.C. The Impact of the Laterality on Radiographic Outcomes of the Bernese Periacetabular Osteotomy. *J. Pers. Med.* **2022**, *12*, 1072. https://doi.org/10.3390/jpm12071072

Academic Editor: Raimund Winter

Received: 24 March 2022
Accepted: 28 June 2022
Published: 29 June 2022

Publisher's Note: MDPI stays neutral with regard to jurisdictional claims in published maps and institutional affiliations.

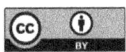

Copyright: © 2022 by the authors. Licensee MDPI, Basel, Switzerland. This article is an open access article distributed under the terms and conditions of the Creative Commons Attribution (CC BY) license (https:// creativecommons.org/licenses/by/ 4.0/).

Abstract: The purpose of this study was to compare the pre and postoperative radiographic findings and analyze the complication rate with respect to the laterality in periacetabular osteotomy in right-handed surgeons. Satisfaction rate and radiographic findings were prospectively collected between 2017 and 2019 and retrospectively reviewed. For analysis, all measurements of the CT scans were performed by a musculoskeletal fellowship-trained radiologist. Complications were classified into two categories: perioperative or postoperative. All surgeries were performed by three right-hand dominant hip surgeons. A total of 41 dysplastic hips (25 right and 16 left hips) in 33 patients were included. Postoperatively, a significantly lower acetabular index angle on the left side was observed at -2.6 ± 4.3 as compared to the right side at 1.6 ± 6.5 ($p < 0.05$). The change in Center edge (CE) angle was significantly lower for the left side $13.7 \pm 5.5°$ than on the right side, measured at 18.4 ± 7.3 ($p < 0.001$); however, the overall CE angle was comparable at $38.5 \pm 8.9°$ without any significant difference between the operated hips (left side at $37.8 \pm 6.1°$ versus right side at 39.0 ± 10.3; $p = 0.340$). No significant differences in other radiographic measurements or surgical time were observed. For complications, the right side was more commonly affected, which may also explain a higher satisfaction rate in patients who were operated on the left hip with 92.3%. The change in lateral CE angle was significantly lower for the left side and the right hip seems to be predisposed to complications, which correlate with a lower satisfaction rate in right-handed surgeons.

Keywords: radiography; periacetabular osteotomy; PAO; dysplasia; complication; laterality

1. Introduction

One of the most common causes of secondary osteoarthritis is developmental dysplasia of the hip [1]. To manage the risk of early-onset osteoarthritis, periacetabular osteotomy (PAO) is the method of choice. Initially described by Ganz in the 1980s, the Bernese PAO allows for repositioning the acetabulum to reduce super-lateral acetabular inclination and improve femoral head coverage, thus restoring the joint center [2]. Indications consist of persistent pain, age between 15 and 45 years of age, positive impingement test, good range of motion, lack of severe osteoarthritis (Kellgren–Lawrence score less than 2), crossing-over sign, and presence of center edge (CE) angle less or equal to 25° [3].

Surgeons try to achieve a horizontal acetabular weight-bearing area [4] with PAO while ensuring that the osteotomy sites stay in contact to avoid nonunion. The acetabular inclination (AI) angle should be between 0° and 10°, whereas the CE angle is aimed to be approximately 35° for the best outcome, according to Hartig-Andreasen [5].

The current literature supports the use of PAO for correcting radiographic deformity and improvement in hip function can be inferred by a low total hip arthroplasty (THA) conversion rate between 0 and 17% of cases [6–8]; however, the complication rate can be as high as 37% according to some studies, in part due to the steep learning curve [9,10]. To improve satisfaction, factors other than radiographic angles and indices, such as the presence of an aspherical femoral head, have to be considered [6].

When looking for total hip arthroplasties, an impact of the laterality, as well as surgeon's handedness, was observed, especially in the positioning of the cup [11]. Hereby, an inclination angle of the acetabular component revealed 46.4° on the dominant operated side compared to 43.5° to the non-dominant side [12].

For periacetabular osteotomy, an accurate reorientation of the acetabulum is even more important to avoid osteoarthritis. To our knowledge, no study to date has investigated the laterality as one of the factors in determining the radiographical outcomes.

For PAO, this study analyzes the laterality of surgery on (1) the radiographic outcome, including the positioning of the socket and (2) complication rate.

2. Materials and Methods

A retrospective study was conducted to evaluate the outcomes of consecutive patients undergoing the Bernese periacetabular osteotomy between 2017 and 2019. Inclusion criteria consisted of complete pre and postoperative assessment of patients older than 18 years of age with a minimum follow-up of 6 months. Patients younger than 18 years of age, with incomplete records (such as missing anteroposterior radiography of the hip instead of the pelvis), or with shorter follow-up were excluded.

To undergo surgery, patients have to meet hip dysplasia criteria published by Tannast et al., have no signs of severe radiographic osteoarthritis, and endured consistent hip pain for at least 1 year [13]. This includes a CE angle of below 20°, an AIA (femoral head bony coverage by the acetabulum) of more than 10°, an AHI (difference between the horizontal line connecting both triradiate cartilages (Hilgenreiner line) and the acetabular roofs) of more than 25% or a sharp angle of more than 42°. Borderline hip dysplasia is defined as a CE angle between 20° and 24.9° and a sharp angle between 39° to 42°, respectively; the presence of a crossing-over sign was used.

All surgeries were performed by one of three experienced right-hand dominant hip surgeons. For preoperative diagnostics, a clinical examination including hip range of motion, quality of pain, body weight (kg), height (cm), body mass index (kg/m^2), anteroposterior radiography of the pelvis, axial view of the affected hip, and torsional computed tomography were included. Intraoperatively, the surgical time, anesthesia time, as well as the necessity of blood transfusion, was noted. For postoperative radiographs, an anteroposterior view of the pelvis and axial view of the hip were performed.

Radiographic measurements included the center edge angle, acetabular index angle (AIA), sharp angle, hip lateralization, the centrum-collum-diaphyseal angle (CCD) on the anteroposterior view, and the alpha, as well as beta angle on axial X-ray, were obtained. Additionally, the presence of a crossing-over sign and femoral-acetabular impingement (CAM and/or pincer impingement) were noted.

For torsional computed tomography, a non-contrast CT of the lower extremity on either a 320-row or an 80-row CT scanner (Canon Aquillon ONE Vision Edition/Canon Aquillon PRIME, Canon Medical Systems, Tochigi, Japan) was performed. The scan was performed with 120 kVp tube voltage and automated tube current modulation set at low dose mode with a 0.5 to 1.0 mm slice thickness using iterative reconstruction and a bone kernel. Measurements were performed by a musculoskeletal fellowship-trained radiologist, including an acetabular rotation at the level of the acetabular center. The angle between the target along the posterior and the anterior acetabular edge and a tangent along the right and left sciatic spine was measured. Likewise, the torsions of the femur, tibia, and tibiofemoral torsion were determined again by an image baseline parallel to the inferior image border. The difference between the femoral neck rotation and the rotation of the femoral condyles resulted in femoral torsion. The tibial torsion was obtained as the differences between tibial plateau rotation and the rotation of the upper ankle. Finally, the tibiofemoral rotation was calculated as the difference between the femoral condyle rotation and the tibial plateau rotation. All rotational measurements are illustrated in Figure 1. In addition, Figures 2–5 show two examples of left, respectively, right-sided dysplastic/borderline dysplastic hip before and after surgery.

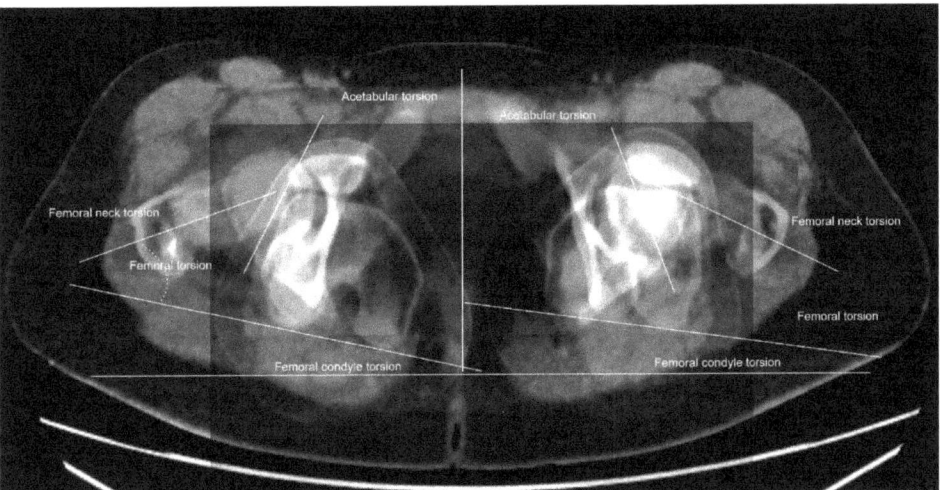

Figure 1. Rotational alignment in a 29-year-old patient with left-sided dysplastic hip: Femoral neck rotation +22°, femoral condyle rotation −24°, femoral rotation +46°, tibial plateau rotation −21°, and femorotibial rotation difference +3°.

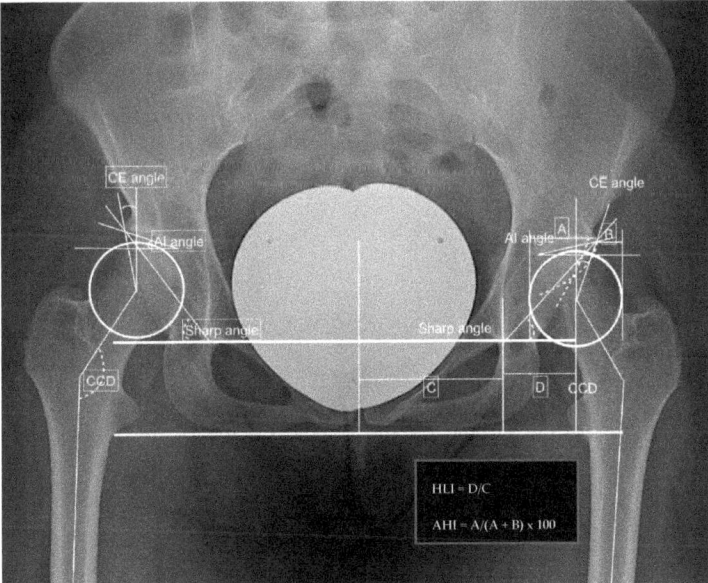

Figure 2. Preoperative findings and measurements performed; left side: CE angle 18.8°, AIA 12.3°, sharp angle 43.9°, hip lateralization 0.54, anterior hip index 73.9, CCD angle 137.4°, and positive crossing-over sign.

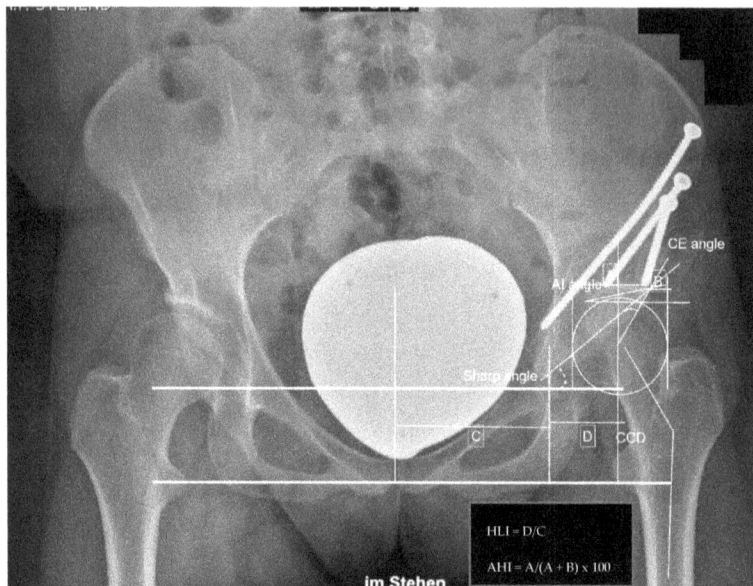

Figure 3. Postoperative measurements after left-sided PAO: CE angle 38.0°, AIA −0.5°, sharp angle 36.5°, hip lateralization 0.56, anterior hip index 91.4, CCD angle 137.4°, and positive crossing-over sign.

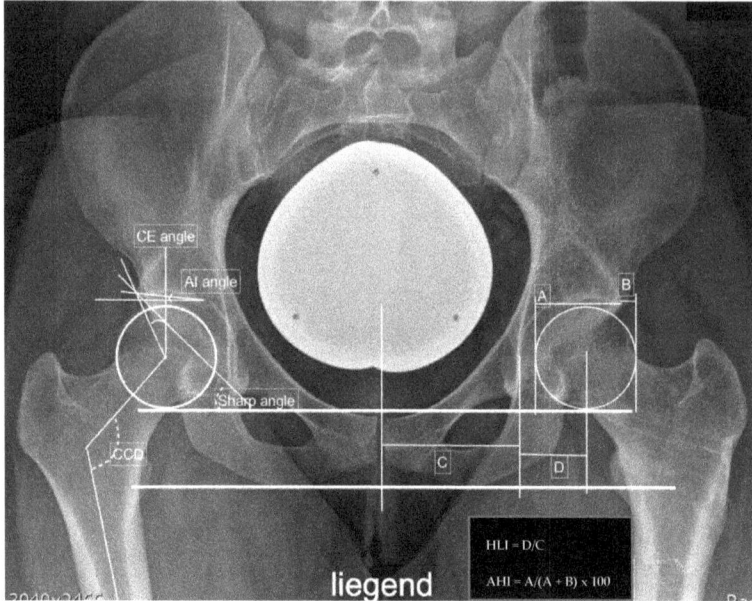

Figure 4. Preoperative measurements in a right-sided borderline dysplastic hip: CE angle 23.4°, AIA 4.9°, sharp angle 40.0°, hip lateralization 0.51, anterior hip index 82.8, and CCD angle 121.0°.

During follow-up, the functional outcome was classified into (1) very satisfied, (2) satisfied, (3) neither satisfied nor dissatisfied, and (4) dissatisfied. The complications were defined as either perioperative, such as bleeding that required blood transfusion, or postoperative complications, such as wound healing issues and postoperative hematoma. In addition, the hardware removal rate related to discomfort was recorded.

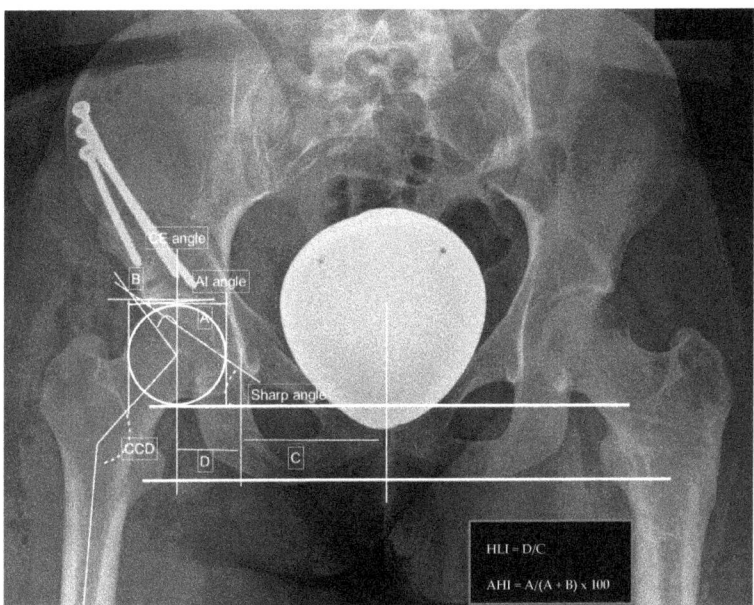

Figure 5. Postoperative measurements after right-sided PAO: CE angle 38.8°, AIA −5.1°, sharp angle 28.0°, hip lateralization 0.57, anterior hip index 90.3, CCD angle 121.0°, and positive crossing-over sign.

For statistical analysis, Microsoft Excel (Version 16.36, Microsoft Corporation, Redmond, WA 98052-6399, USA), IBM® SPSS® Statistics 26 Core System (IBM, Armonk, NY, USA), and Origin Pro 8.0 (OriginLab Cooperation, Northampton, MA 01060, USA) were used. The mean and standard deviation of the mean (SD) are presented for all normally distributed continuous variables. A multivariate Analysis of Variance (ANOVA) T-Test was applied, and level of significances were set to * $p < 0.05$, ** $p < 0.01$, and *** $p < 0.005$. All values are recorded to one decimal place. An a priori power analysis was shown when using conservative estimation to achieve 80% power at a 5% significance level; an effect size of 1.5 can be assumed, requiring 8 subjects (PASS 2008).

3. Results

Between 2017 and 2019, a total of 41 hips in 33 patients were included. Of the 41 hips, 25 right and 16 left hips underwent PAO. The mean age was 28.6 ± 7.4 years without any significant differences between the two groups. The mean age of the left hip group was 29.4 ± 7.7 as compared to the right side at the age of 28.1 ± 7.1 ($p = 0.288$). Females gender consisted of 90.1% of cases with no difference among the two groups (left side 100.0%, right side 80.8%; $p = 0.048$).

Similarly, no differences were observed for height at 169.7 ± 8.3 cm (left side 168.1 ± 7.6 cm, right side 170.7 ± 8.5 cm; $p = 0.178$), body weight at 68.0 ± 11.7 kg (left side 65.6 ± 9.3 kg, right side 69.6 ± 12.7 kg; $p = 0.159$), and body mass index at 23.6 ± 3.8 kg/m² (left side 23.5 ± 3.1 kg/m², right side 69.6 ± 12.7 kg/m²; $p = 0.450$). In our cohort, borderline dysplastic hips were diagnosed in 68.3% of patients (left hip group with 75.0%, $n = 12/16$; right hip group with 64.0% $n = 16/25$; $p = 0.236$). Depression was observed in seven cases (17.1%, $n = 7/41$), which were equally distributed between the two groups: left side at 18.8% ($n = 3/16$) and right side at 16.0% ($n = 4/25$). Other comorbidities included asthma bronchiale in two cases ($n = 2/41$, 4.9%, one in each group). There is one Crohn's disease patient in the left hip group

(n = 1/16) and one case of mitral regurgitation in the right hip group (n = 1/25). For fixation of the socket, screws were used in 85.4% (n = 35/41, left hip group 87.5%, n = 14/16, respectively, right hip group 84.0%, n = 21/25) of cases. In the remaining cases k-wires were used for fixation. All demographics are illustrated in Table 1.

Table 1. Demographics of included patients and significance between the two groups.

Observation	Overall	Left Hip	Right Hip	p-Value
Numbers (%)	41 (100)	16 (39.0)	25 (61.0)	
Dysplastic hips (%)	13 (31.7)	4 (25.0)	9 (36.0)	0.236
Age (mean age)	28.6 ± 7.4	29.4 ± 7.7	28.1 ± 7.1	0.288
Follow up in days	267.5 ± 208.5	222.7 ± 251.0	296.7 ± 169.0	0.149
Gender (female) n (%)	37 (90.1)	16 (100)	21 (80.8)	0.048
Body height (cm)	169.7 ± 8.3	168.1 ± 7.6	170.7 ± 8.5	0.178
Body weight (kg)	68.0 ± 11.7	65.6 ± 9.3	69.6 ± 12.7	0.159
Body mass index (kg/m^2)	23.6 ± 3.8	23.5 ± 3.1	23.7 ± 4.2	0.450
Mental disorders, Depression n (%)	7 (17.1)	3 (18.8)	4 (16.0)	0.412
Fixation (screws) n (%)	35 (85.4)	14 (87.5)	21 (84.0)	0.382

For follow-up, the mean was 267.5 ± 208.5 days with no significant difference between the two groups (left side 222.7 ± 251.0 days versus 296.7 ± 169.0 days; p = 0.149). In all patients, the union was observed at their final follow-up.

Preoperatively, significant differences between the two groups were observed for CE angle and alpha angle on radiography. The CE angle was 22.0 ± 6.2° overall (left group 24.1 ± 5.2° versus right group 20.7 ± 6.5°; p = 0.045). The alpha angle was 100.7 ± 10.7 overall (left group 97.0 ± 9.5° versus right group 103.4 ± 10.7; p = 0.034). The rotational alignment revealed no significant differences between the groups preoperatively. The findings are summarized in Table 2.

Table 2. Rotational alignment of the lower extremity before surgery.

Rotational Values	Overall	Left Hip	Right Hip	p-Value
Acetabular torsion (°)	18.8 ± 6.9	18.8 ± 6.9	19.3 ± 5.6	0.388
Femoral torsion (°)	30.5 ± 12.9	27.7 ± 14.1	13.3 ± 18.8	0.139
Tibial torsion (°)	37.4 ± 11.0	37.0 ± 7.6	41.8 ± 8.8	0.433
Femorotibial torsion (°)	6.2 ± 5.4	−6.6 ± 11.1	7.8 ± 3.6	0.082

After surgery, a significant difference was observed for the acetabular index angle (AIA) with a mean of −0.02 ± 6.1 and a p-value of 0.016 (left side −2.6 ± 4.3 compared to 1.6 ± 6.5 on the right side).

When comparing the radiographic changes before to after the periacetabular osteotomy, significant differences were noted for all parameters measured except the beta angle, which has a p-value of 0.210. Likewise, similar findings were observed for the individual groups. The left side changed significantly in all radiographic measurements except the CCD, alpha, and beta angle with p-values of 0.179, 0.241, and 0.163, respectively. For the right side, no significant differences were observed for the CCD and beta angle with p-values of 0.081 and 0.411, respectively (see Table 3).

Although significant differences were observed in all cases, the positioning of the left side was more accurate to the estimated CE-angle of approximately 35°. All measurements are illustrated in Table 3 and changes in radiographic parameters are summarized in Table 4.

Table 3. Radiographic findings pre and postoperatively include significant differences between the individual groups. (Bold values denote statistical significance).

X-ray Measurements	Preoperatively				Postoperatively				Difference
	Overall	Left Hip	Right Hip	p-Value	Overall	Left Hip	Right Hip	p-Value	p-Value
CE angle (°)	22.0 ± 6.2	24.1 ± 5.2	20.7 ± 6.5	**0.045**	38.5 ± 8.9	37.8 ± 6.1	39.0 ± 10.3	0.340	**<0.001**
AIA (°)	11.7 ± 5.7	10.6 ± 4.4	12.4 ± 6.3	0.172	−0.02 ± 6.1	−2.6 ± 4.3	1.6 ± 6.5	**0.016**	**<0.001**
Sharp angle (°)	42.9 ± 3.8	41.7 ± 3.3	43.6 ± 3.9	0.069	30.1 ± 5.0	29.3 ± 5.9	30.7 ± 4.3	0.194	**<0.001**
Hip lateralization	0.56 ± 0.07	0.55 ± 0.06	0.56 ± 0.07	0.363	0.62 ± 0.07	0.60 ± 0.05	0.62 ± 0.09	0.179	**<0.001**
Anterior hip index	75.5 ± 7.5	77.4 ± 6.4	74.3 ± 7.8	0.100	89.7 ± 6.8	90.8 ± 6.2	89.1 ± 7.0	0.229	**<0.001**
CCD angle (°)	134.1 ± 6.0	133.0 ± 4.8	134.8 ± 6.5	0.182	136.5 ± 6.8	134.6 ± 4.9	137.7 ± 7.5	0.083	**0.047**
CAM FAI n (%)	17 (41.5)	6 (37.5)	11 (44.0)	0.345					
Pincer FAI	2 (4.9)	0 (0)	2 (8.0)	0.128					
Crossing-over sign	14 (34.1)	5 (31.3)	9 (36.0)	0.381					
Kellgren-Lawrence score 0	25 (61.0)	10 (62.5)	15 (60.0)	0.294					
Kellgren-Lawrence score 1	14 (34.1)	6 (37.5)	8 (32.0)						
Kellgren-Lawrence score 2	2 (4.9)	0 (0)	2 (8.0)						
Alpha angle (°)	100.7 ± 10.7	97.0 ± 9.5	103.4 ± 10.7	**0.034**	90.9 ± 12.9	92.1 ± 17.8	90.4 ± 9.9	0.422	**0.005**
Beta angle (°)	57.5 ± 7.4	56.5 ± 7.0	58.3 ± 7.6	0.234	59.4 ± 5.7	60.4 ± 4.4	59.0 ± 6.2	0.355	0.210

Table 4. Changes in radiographic parameters between the two groups. (Bold values denote statistical significance).

X-ray Measurements	Change			
	Overall	Left Hip	Right Hip	p-Value
CE angle (°)	16.6 ± 7.1	13.7 ± 5.5	18.4 ± 7.3	**0.021**
AIA (°)	−11.7 ± 5.7	−13.2 ± 6.0	−10.7 ± 5.2	0.093
Sharp angle (°)	−12.7 ± 4.0	−12.5 ± 4.7	−12.9 ± 3.5	0.381
Hip lateralization	0.06 ± 0.06	0.05 ± 0.05	0.06 ± 0.06	0.213
Anterior hip index	14.2 ± 5.2	13.4 ± 5.0	14.8 ± 5.2	0.195
Alpha angle (°)	−3.6 ± 30.3	−0.5 ± 16.5	−4.9 ± 34.24	0.412
Beta angle (°)	4.7 ± 18.5	2.3 ± 6.1	5.7 ± 21.4	0.386

For fixation of the acetabular fragment, screws were used in 85.4% of cases (left side n = 14/16, 87.5% versus right side n = 21/25, 84.0%, p = 0.382). The mean surgical time was 89 ± 32 min with no significant differences (left group 85 ± 22 min versus 91 ± 37 min, p = 0.290). The mean anesthesia time was 148 ± 41 min (left side 143 ± 27 min compared to 152 ± 47 min, p = 0.260).

Due to intraoperative bleeding, transfusion was required in seven cases (n = 7/41, 17.1%). Of this cohort, the right hip was involved in six cases (n = 6/25, 24.0% compared to n = 1/16, 6.3%, p = 0.07). Other complications included hypesthesia of the lateral cutaneous femoral nerve in 37 cases (n = 37/41, 90.2%, left side n = 14/16, 87.5% versus right side n = 22/25, 88.0%, p = 0.482); one common peroneal nerve palsy and one postoperative infection that required debridement (n = 1/25, 4.0%). Furthermore, two cases of loss of implant fixation were observed, with one in each group (4.9%, left side n = 1/16, 6.3% compared to the right side n = 1/25, 4.0%, p = 0.376). Hardware removal was performed in nine right hips and one left hip due to irritation. No significances were observed (p = 0.161) between groups for satisfaction score, with a total of 39.0% of patients who were very satisfied, 22% reporting satisfied, 7.3% reporting neither satisfied nor dissatisfied, and 17.1% reporting dissatisfied. Patients who underwent right-sided PAO were dissatisfied at a rate of 24.0% (n = 6/25) as compared to 6.3% (n = 1/16) (p = 0.25). All complications are listed in Table 5.

Eight female patients underwent bilateral periacetabular osteotomy by the same surgeon, with significant differences for postoperative AIA and anterior hip index. There was also trending toward significance for all other radiographic measurements. All findings are summarized in Table 6.

Table 5. Complication rate after periacetabular osteotomy. (Bold values denote statistical significance).

Complications	Overall	Left Side	Right Side	p-Value
Transfusion (%)	7 (17.1)	1 (6.3)	6 (24.0)	0.07
Hypesthesia of lateral cutaneous femoral nerve (%)	37 (90.2)	14 (87.5)	22 (88.0)	0.482
Implant migration (%)	2 (4.9)	1 (6.3)	1 (4.0)	0.376
Peroneal communis nerve palsy (%)	1 (2.4)	0 (0)	1 (4.0)	**<0.001**
Wound infection (%)	1 (2.4)	0 (0)	1 (4.0)	**<0.001**
Hardware removal (%)	10 (24.4)	1 (6.3)	9 (36.0)	**0.015**

Table 6. Findings in patients who underwent bilateral PAO. (Bold values denote statistical significance).

Demographic Data	Overall				Left Hip	Right Hip			p-Value
Age (mean age)	29.1 ± 6.9				28.9 ± 6.9	29.3 ± 6.9			0.460
Follow up in days	303.6 ± 243.2				271.4 ± 312.7	335.9 ± 135.7			0.312
Body height (cm)	167.7 ± 6.1				167.8 ± 6.2	167.6 ± 6.1			0.485
Body weight (kg)	67.7 ± 7.2				68.1 ± 7.6	67.3 ± 6.7			0.411
Body mass index (kg/m^2)	24.1 ± 2.8				24.3 ± 2.9	24.0 ± 2.7			0.432
Comparison	Preoperatively				Postoperatively				Difference
	Overall	Left Hip	Right Hip	p-Value	Overall	Left Hip	Right Hip	p-Value	p-Value
CE angle (°)	20.7 ± 5.8	23.0 ± 5.0	18.4 ± 5.6	0.063	39.2 ± 8.6	38.7 ± 5.0	39.8 ± 11.0	0.413	**<0.001**
AIA (°)	13.6 ± 4.4	11.8 ± 4.0	15.4 ± 3.9	0.056	−0.11 ± 4.8	−2.8 ± 4.0	2.6 ± 4.0	**0.013**	**<0.001**
Sharp angle (°)	43.1 ± 4.2	41.5 ± 3.3	44.7 ± 4.4	0.072	30.1 ± 4.5	28.3 ± 4.0	31.9 ± 4.2	0.060	**<0.001**
Hip lateralization	0.556 ± 0.07	0.56 ± 0.08	0.55 ± 0.06	0.386	0.59 ± 0.05	0.60 ± 0.04	0.59 ± 0.05	0.384	**0.043**
Anterior hip index	73.7 ± 6.4	76.6 ± 5.9	70.8 ± 5.5	**0.039**	90.1 ± 5.7	92.7 ± 4.9	87.5 ± 5.2	**0.037**	**<0.001**
Change in Radiographic Parameters									
CE angle (°)	18.5 ± 6.9				15.7 ± 4.7	21.3 ± 7.5			0.057
AIA (°)	−13.7 ± 5.3				−14.6 ± 5.9	−12.8 ± 4.5			0.268
Sharp angle (°)	−13.0 ± 3.8				−13.2 ± 3.7	−12.8 ± 3.9			0.416
Hip lateralization	0.04 ± 0.06				0.04 ± 0.05	0.04 ± 0.07			0.452
Anterior hip index	16.4 ± 4.2				16.1 ± 4.9	16.7 ± 3.2			0.396
Complications									
Transfusion (%)	2 (12.5)				0 (0)	2 (25.0)			0.074
Hypesthesia of lateral cutaneous femoral nerve (%)	16 (100)				8 (100)	8 (100)			1.000
Implant migration (%)	2 (12.5)				1 (12.5)	1 (12.5)			1.000
Hardware removal (%)	2 (12.5)				0 (0)	2 (25)			0.074
Operative Time									
Surgical time (min)	93 ± 36				89 ± 25	97 ± 44			0.340
Anaesthesia time (min)	152 ± 46				147 ± 31	157 ± 57			0.355

4. Discussion

This study analyses the impact of the laterality on outcomes following PAO. Our patient cohort suggests that the laterality in PAO has an impact on the degree of correction as well as complication rate. Hereby, the right hip PAO is at higher risk for complications, including intraoperative bleeding ($p = 0.07$) or others ($p = 0.482$); however, without any significance. In addition, the CE angle after positioning of the acetabular fragment is slightly higher compared to the left side, with a significant difference in AIA ($p = 0.016$) and a change in CE angle ($p = 0.021$). In our series, right hip PAO has a higher rate of wound infection, peroneal nerve palsy, and transfusion. This may also explain the lower satisfaction rate in patients who underwent right-sided PAO.

The Bernese periacetabular osteotomy is a well-established method to manage the risk of osteoarthritis. The surgical techniques used are described in Appendix A. Typically, the mean change in acetabular inclination (sharp angle) ranges from 4.5° to 25.9°, leading to a change in lateral CE angle from 20° to 44° and a medial translation of the hip center from 5 mm to 10 mm. This is confirmed by our study with a change in the sharp angle of 12.7 ± 4.0°, whereas our change in CE angle was rather low with a change of 16.6 ± 7.1°. Clinically, pain relief can be observed in short and midterm follow-ups as well as improvement in Harris hip score; however, improvement in hip function was not predictable. Major complications occurred in 6% to 37% of cases, including heterotopic ossifications, wound hematomas, nerve palsies, intraarticular osteotomies, loss of fixation, and malreductions [7,14]. In our cohort, the complication rate, including loss of implant fixation, was 4.9%, infection was 4.0%, peroneal palsy was 4.0%, and the necessity of transfusion was 17.1%. When looking for conversion to hip arthroplasty after PAO, this is described to be 96.1% for 5 years, 91.3% for 10 years, 85.0% for 15 years, and 67.6% for 20 years in one meta-analysis [15].

The conversion rate to total hip arthroplasty ranges from 0% to 17%. [8,14] Although no recommendations for optimal femoral coverage can be found, Hartig-Andreasen described that CE angle improvements less than 30° or more than 40° is a risk factor for conversion to total hip arthroplasty [5]. Overcorrection of the acetabulum may increase the dissatisfaction rate and risk of pincer femoro-acetabular impingement (FAI) syndrome as well as osteoarthritis. It is also possible to develop pincer FAI syndrome in postoperative CE angle over 46° [16]. Other radiographic measurements described by Tannast et al. for over-covered hips included a lateral center edge angle between 34° and 39° and an acetabular index between −7° to 2° in non-operated hips. The sharp angle was found to be normal between 38° to 42° and 34° to 37° for over-coverage [13].

For the laterality and surgeon handedness, Moloney et al. were among the first to describe that it may have an impact on surgical outcome [17]. For total hip arthroplasty using the lateral approach, significant differences were observed for the cup inclination angles when a surgeon is operating on the side of the dominant hand; however, the differences may not be clinically significant [12].

This study is limited by small sample size and lack of a case match control arm. In addition to the inclination angle, surgeons are more likely to use a larger ante version on the non-dominant hip ($p = 0.043$). Furthermore, the authors reported a more accurate result when operating on their dominant side [11]. The interplay between surgeon handedness and laterality of the hip undergoing surgery can result in lower abduction and less combined Lewinnek outliers [18].

A possible explanation for the differences in laterality may result from the technique used for reorientation of the osteotomized acetabular fragment, such as a supra-acetabular Schanz screw, until optimal femoral coverage is obtained. Alternatively, a laminar spreader can be used to re-orientate the acetabular fragment, which allows finer adjustment. Once the most suitable position is found, fixation is performed using either a combination of K-wires or screws. Since the surgeon aims for an increased CE angle by pushing the fragment downwards, this may explain the higher CE angle for the dominant right hip for right-handed surgeons. Other factors that may influence the final position are the necessity for bony contact to allow for healing as well as soft tissue constraints. To assess the correction of the acetabulum more accurately, an intraoperative anteroposterior pelvic radiograph could be obtained instead of fluoroscopy. This allows comparing the preoperative imaging with the intraoperative findings better.

In our cohort, no significant differences in demographics between the two groups were found. Preoperatively, CE angles were significantly higher in the left hips compared to the right one ($p = 0.045$). This may result from more right leg dominant patients correlated with more severe symptoms. Postoperatively, higher CE angles were found on the right hip ($39.0 \pm 10.3°$) with significantly higher AIA of $1.6 \pm 6.5°$. Other trends towards significance were observed for the sharp angle and hip lateralization. When considering Hartig-Andreasen et al.'s recommendations, the left hip seems to have better radiographic parameters postoperatively in right-hand dominant surgeons [5]. In addition, a higher complication rate was observed for the right hip, including more instances of transfusion and a significantly higher rate for peroneal communis nerve palsy. This may also explain the higher numbers of dissatisfied patients in the right hip group.

This study has limitations. Periacetabular osteotomy is a challenging surgery that only a few highly specialized surgeons perform—all of them are right dominant at our center [19,20]. The cohort was rather small and all PAOs were performed by three surgeons; however, the same technique was used since all were trained by the same senior surgeon. In addition, this is a retrospective study with no control arm. Although the complication number was small and the radiographic differences were small, the a priori power analysis showed that at least eight patients are required. A possible explanation for the higher satisfaction in left-sided hips may result from a pivotal reason. Hereby, a higher degree of dysplasia does not necessarily mean a lower CE angle but also a higher acetabular deformity. This could lead to a more challenging periacetabular osteotomy. Lastly, this study also did not look at inter-surgeon variation in technique and fixation method. For the radiographic measurements, it must be mentioned that projection of the radiographs can also affect angulation, therefore impacting our analysis. To minimize the bias of rotation deformity in all patients, a rotational CT was performed. Although we only included patients with a minimum follow-up of 6 months and union was observed in all cases, longer follow-up is needed to investigate the functional outcome.

5. Conclusions

In our patient cohort, it appears that right side PAO is at risk for a higher rate of complications. This depends not only on the laterality but also on many factors, including but not limited to surgical technique, fixation method, and patient anatomy. We recommend further studies to evaluate the surgeon handedness on a prospective basis with a matched control arm.

Author Contributions: Conceptualization, C.Y.W.H. and H.C.B.; methodology, C.Y.W.H., H.C.B., F.G.; software, C.Y.W.H. and H.C.B.; validation, C.Y.W.H., F.G. and H.C.B.; formal analysis, C.Y.W.H. and H.C.B.; investigation, C.Y.W.H., C.H.W. and H.C.B.; resources, C.P., S.H.; data curation, C.Y.W.H. and H.C.B.; writing—original draft preparation, C.Y.W.H., C.H.W., F.G., C.P., S.H. and H.C.B.; writing—review and editing, C.Y.W.H., C.H.W., F.G., C.P., S.H. and H.C.B.; visualization, H.C.B. and C.P.; supervision, C.P., H.C.B.; project administration, H.C.B. All authors have read and agreed to the published version of the manuscript.

Funding: This research received no external funding.

Institutional Review Board Statement: The study was conducted in accordance with the Declaration of Helsinki, and approved by the Institutional Review Board of the Charite Berlin, Germany (protocol code EA4_201_19 and 12 November 2019).

Informed Consent Statement: Patient consent was waived due to the retrospective design.

Data Availability Statement: Not applicable.

Acknowledgments: We acknowledge support from the German Research Foundation (DFG) and the Open Access Publication Funds of Charité—Universitätsmedizin Berlin.

Conflicts of Interest: The authors declare no conflict of interest.

Appendix A

For the periacetabular osteotomy, patients are placed in a supine position on a radiolucent table and the ipsilateral arm is placed across the chest. The operated hip is prepped and draped to visualize the iliac crest and hemipelvis. Hereby, the ipsilateral foot should be included.

A modified Smith–Petersen approach with an incision up to the iliac crest is performed. The fascia over the tensor is incised and the abductor muscles are preserved as well as the lateral femoral cutaneous nerve should be protected proximally around the anterior superior iliac spine. Now the tensor fascial muscle is retracted laterally, and the external oblique muscle is dissected off the iliac crest, which allows accessing the inner pelvis. Distally the rectus abdominal muscle is retracted from the anterior inferior iliac spine following dissection of the iliocapsularis muscle off the anterior hip capsule, allowing the palpation of the calcar femoris. For medial dissection, the quadrilateral surface and pubic root are visualized.

The periacetabular osteotomy is performed with an osteotome beginning with the inferior retro-acetabular osteotomy from the infracotyloid groove towards the middle of the ischial spine. The ischial osteotomy is incomplete, with a depth of about 2.5 cm. After retracting the iliopsoas muscle and femoral neurovascular bundle medially, the ramus pubis is cut. Hereby, the osteotome should exit the medial to the obturator nerve. In a further stage, the iliac osteotomy is performed while preserving the superior gluteal artery and vascular arcade supplying the acetabulum. The medial cortex is cut first, followed by the posterior column at an angle of 120 degrees subchondrally.

To confirm the osteotomy, fluoroscopy is used. Now a Laminar spreader and a Schanz screw (5.0 mm) are placed in the superior aspect of the mobile fragment and used for reorientation; therefore, an inwards turn up to an adequate reorientation by internal rotation, forward tilt/extension, and medial translation. The mobile fragment is fixated temporarily using K-wires. The correction is confirmed with an image intensifier again to evaluate the radiographic measurements following definite fixation with K-wires or several 3.5 mm/4.5 mm fully threaded screws. After irrigation and a final hemostasis, the wound is closed in layers [8,19,20].

References

1. Aronson, J. Osteoarthritis of the young adult hip: Etiology and treatment. *Instr. Course Lect.* **1986**, *35*, 119–128. [PubMed]
2. Leunig, M.; Siebenrock, K.A.; Ganz, R. Rationale of periacetabular osteotomy and background work. *J. Bone Jt. Surg.* **2001**, *83*, 438. [CrossRef]
3. Jakobsen, S.S.; Overgaard, S.; Søballe, K.; Ovesen, O.; Mygind-Klavsen, B.; Dippmann, C.A.; Jensen, M.U.; Stürup, J.; Retpen, J. The interface between periacetabular osteotomy, hip arthroscopy and total hip arthroplasty in the young adult hip. *EFORT Open Rev.* **2018**, *3*, 408–417. [CrossRef] [PubMed]
4. Hayashi, S.; Hashimoto, S.; Matsumoto, T.; Takayama, K.; Kamenaga, T.; Niikura, T.; Kuroda, R. Overcorrection of the acetabular roof angle or anterior center-edge angle may cause decrease of range of motion after curved periacetabular osteotomy. *J. Hip Preserv. Surg.* **2020**, *7*, 583–590. [CrossRef] [PubMed]
5. Hartig-Andreasen, C.; Troelsen, A.; Thillemann, T.M.; Søballe, K. What factors predict failure 4 to 12 years after periacetabular osteotomy? *Clin. Orthop. Relat. Res.* **2012**, *470*, 2978–2987. [CrossRef] [PubMed]
6. Clohisy, J.C.; Schutz, A.L.; St. John, L.; Schoenecker, P.L.; Wright, R.W. Periacetabular Osteotomy: A Systematic Literature Review. *Clin. Orthop. Relat. Res.* **2009**, *467*, 2041–2052. [CrossRef] [PubMed]
7. Biedermann, R.; Donnan, L.; Gabriel, A.; Wachter, R.; Krismer, M.; Behensky, H. Complications and patient satisfaction after periacetabular pelvic osteotomy. *Int. Orthop.* **2007**, *32*, 611–617. [CrossRef] [PubMed]
8. Siebenrock, K.A.; Scholl, E.; Lottenbach, M.; Ganz, R. Bernese periacetabular osteotomy. *Clin. Orthop. Relat. Res.* **1999**, 9–20. [CrossRef]
9. Davey, J.P.; Santore, R.F. Complications of Periacetabular Osteotomy. *Clin. Orthop. Relat. Res.* **1999**, *363*, 33–37. [CrossRef]
10. Mayo, K.A.; Trumble, S.J.; Mast, J.W. Results of Periacetabular Osteotomy in Patients with Previous Surgery for Hip Dysplasia. *Clin. Orthop. Relat. Res.* **1999**, *363*, 73–80. [CrossRef]
11. Kong, X.; Yang, M.; Li, X.; Ni, M.; Zhang, G.; Chen, J.; Chai, W. Impact of surgeon handedness in manual and robot-assisted total hip arthroplasty. *J. Orthop. Surg. Res.* **2020**, *15*, 159. [CrossRef]
12. Pennington, N.; Redmond, A.; Stewart, T.; Stone, M. The impact of surgeon handedness in total hip replacement. *Ann. R. Coll. Surg. Engl.* **2014**, *96*, 437–441. [CrossRef] [PubMed]
13. Tannast, M.; Hanke, M.S.; Zheng, G.; Steppacher, S.D.; Siebenrock, K.A. What are the radiographic reference values for acetabular under- and overcoverage? *Clin. Orthop. Relat. Res.* **2015**, *473*, 1234–1246. [CrossRef] [PubMed]
14. Clohisy, J.C.; Barrett, S.E.; Gordon, J.E.; Delgado, E.; Schoenecker, P.L. Periacetabular osteotomy for the treatment of severe acetabular dysplasia. *J. Bone Jt. Surg.* **2005**, *87*, 254–259. [CrossRef] [PubMed]
15. Ahmad, S.S.; Giebel, G.M.; Perka, C.; Meller, S.; Pumberger, M.; Hardt, S.; Stöckle, U.; Konrads, C. Survival of the dysplastic hip after periacetabular osteotomy: A meta-analysis. *HIP Int.* **2021**, 11207000211048425. [CrossRef]
16. Imai, H.; Kamada, T.; Takeba, J.; Shiraishi, Y.; Mashima, N.; Miura, H. Anterior coverage after eccentric rotational acetabular osteotomy for the treatment of developmental dysplasia of the hip. *J. Orthop. Sci.* **2014**, *19*, 762–769. [CrossRef]
17. Moloney, D.; Bishay, M.; Ivory, J.; Pozo, J. Failure of the sliding hip screw in the treatment of femoral neck fractures: 'Left-handed surgeons for left-sided hips'. *Injury* **1994**, *25*, SB9–SB13. [CrossRef]
18. Crawford, D.A.; Adams, J.B.; Hobbs, G.R.; Lombardi, A.J.V.; Berend, K.R. Surgical Approach and Hip Laterality Affect Accuracy of Acetabular Component Placement in Primary Total Hip Arthroplasty. *Surg. Technol. Int.* **2019**, *35*, 377–385. [PubMed]

19. Siebenrock, K.A.; Leunig, M.; Ganz, R. Periacetabular osteotomy: The Bernese experience. *Instr. Course Lect.* **2001**, *50*, 239–245. [CrossRef]
20. Kamath, A.F. Bernese periacetabular osteotomy for hip dysplasia: Surgical technique and indications. *World J. Orthop.* **2016**, *7*, 280–286. [CrossRef]

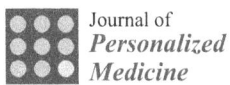

Article

HR-pQCT for the Evaluation of Muscle Quality and Intramuscular Fat Infiltration in Ageing Skeletal Muscle

Simon Kwoon-Ho Chow [1,*], Marloes van Mourik [2], Vivian Wing-Yin Hung [1], Ning Zhang [1], Michelle Meng-Chen Li [1], Ronald Man-Yeung Wong [1], Kwok-Sui Leung [1] and Wing-Hoi Cheung [1]

[1] Musculoskeletal Research Laboratory, Bone Quality and Health Centre,
Department of Orthopaedics and Traumatology, The Chinese University of Hong Kong, Hong Kong;
vivi@ort.cuhk.edu.hk (V.W.-Y.H.); ningzzz@stanford.edu (N.Z.); mclimichelle@link.cuhk.edu.hk (M.M.-C.L.);
ronald.wong@cuhk.edu.hk (R.M.-Y.W.); ksleung@cuhk.edu.hk (K.-S.L.); louis@ort.cuhk.edu.hk (W.-H.C.)
[2] Orthopaedic Biomechanics, Department of Biomedical Engineering, Eindhoven University of Technology,
5600 MB Eindhoven, The Netherlands; m.v.mourik@tue.nl
* Correspondence: skhchow@link.cuhk.edu.hk; Tel.: +852-3505-1559

Abstract: Myosteatosis is the infiltration of fat in skeletal muscle during the onset of sarcopenia. The quantification of intramuscular adipose tissue (IMAT) can be a feasible imaging modality for the clinical assessment of myosteatosis, important for the early identification of sarcopenia patients and timely intervention decisions. There is currently no standardized method or consensus for such an application. The aim of this study was to develop a method for the detection and analysis of IMAT in clinical HR-pQCT images of the distal tibia to evaluate skeletal muscle during the ageing process, validated with animal and clinical experimentation. A pre-clinical model of ovariectomized (OVX) rats with known intramuscular fat infiltration was used, where gastrocnemii were scanned by micro-computed tomography (micro-CT) at an 8.4 µm isotropic voxel size, and the images were analyzed using our modified IMAT analysis protocol. IMAT, muscle density (MD), and muscle volume (MV) were compared with SHAM controls validated with Oil-red-O (ORO) staining. Furthermore, the segmentation and IMAT evaluation method was applied to 30 human subjects at ages from 18 to 81 (mean = 47.3 ± 19.2). Muscle-related parameters were analyzed with functional outcomes. In the animal model, the micro-CT adipose tissue-related parameter of IMAT% segmented at −600 HU to 100 HU was shown to strongly associate with the ORO-positively stained area (r = 0.898, p = 0.002). For the human subjects, at an adjusted threshold of −600 to −20 HU, moderate positive correlations were found between MV and MD (r = 0.642, p < 0.001), and between MV and IMAT volume (r = 0.618, p < 0.01). Moderate negative correlations were detected between MD and IMAT% (r = −0.640, p < 0.001). Strong and moderate associations were found between age and MD (r = 0.763, p < 0.01), and age and IMAT (r = 0.559, p < 0.01). There was also a strong correlation between IMAT% and chair rise time (r = 0.671, p < 0.01). The proposed HR-pQCT evaluation protocol for intramuscular adipose-tissue produced MD and IMAT results that were associated with age and physical performance measures, and were of good predictive value for the progression of myosteatosis or sarcopenia. The protocol was also validated on animal skeletal muscle samples that showed a good representation of histological lipid content with positive correlations, further supporting the clinical application for the rapid evaluation of muscle quality and objective quantification of skeletal muscle at the peripheral for sarcopenia assessment.

Keywords: intramuscular infiltration; sarcopenia; HR-pQCT; aged skeletal muscle; animal model

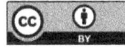

1. Introduction

Sarcopenia is a disease characterized by the progressive loss of skeletal muscle mass and strength [1], which is highly associated with unintentional fall events and fragility fractures in older people [2]. The early detection of sarcopenia would enable personalized treatment decisions for the prevention of fragility fracture. Myosteatosis is the infiltration of fat in skeletal muscle during sarcopenia onset [1,3] with the overall volume of muscle remaining unchanged and the decrease in lean muscle, resulting in an unnoticeable loss in muscle strength and eventually dynapenia (i.e., loss of muscle strength). Delmonico et al. reported that 35.5% to 74.6% of intermuscular fat increase was detected in men aged 70 to 79 in 5 years' time, while a 16.8% to 50.0% increase was detected in women. The fat tissue content within skeletal muscle was also found to be associated negatively with muscle strength in elderly people [4]. These observations are also well supported by a sarcopenic animal model showing that increased intramuscular fat infiltration has direct consequences on muscle strength and physical performance [5]. The exact mechanism that leads to myosteatosis is not fully understood; however, it is believed that disuse, sex steroid depletion, and altered leptin signaling are associated with lipid accumulation in elderly people. Furthermore, it is considered as one of the pathological factors of sarcopenia [6–8], affecting approximately 10% of both males and females in the world [9], leading to poor balancing abilities and a substantial increase in fall risks and rates of fragility fracture (to as much as 1.87 times higher) [10,11].

The imaging and quantification of intramuscular adipose tissue (IMAT) are therefore important to study and understand this factor during skeletal muscle ageing. Various advancements in imaging modalities have made this task possible [12]. Magnetic resonance imaging (MRI) [13,14] and computed tomography (CT) [15,16] are effective gold standards to accurately discriminate adipose tissue from skeletal muscles. However, the clinical application of these imaging techniques are technically limited by the lack of a standardized evaluation protocol [17] and practically limited by its availability and long waiting time at various hospital settings [18]. Alternatively, dual energy absorptiometry (DXA) and bioimpedance analysis (BIA) are suggested as alternatives to quantitatively estimate whole body lean and fat muscle contents [6,19]. However, the resolution of these techniques is limited by their insufficient resolving power to discriminate IMAT.

High-resolution peripheral quantitative computed tomography (HR-pQCT) is an advanced method of evaluating microstructures of the bone [20–22] or muscle at resolutions of up to 41 microns with an effective radiation dose of less than 5 µSv per scan as compared to 50–150 µSv per chest X-ray. HR-pQCT is able to evaluate soft tissues and discriminate adipose tissues from lean skeletal muscles to evaluate a number of parameters important for the estimation of adipose tissues in the region of interest. These parameters include muscle density (MD) and inter- or intramuscular adipose tissue (IMAT), important for the assessment of muscle quality. Furthermore, the HR-pQCT also has the advantage of generating three-dimensional volumetric reconstructions in a relatively short scanning time compared to DXA and BIA. Therefore, it is suggested that HR-pQCT is a feasible method for the evaluation of muscle quality and intramuscular fat infiltration during the progression of sarcopenia. Here, we describe the application of a method for the detection and analysis of intramuscular adipose tissue (IMAT) in clinical HR-pQCT images, to supplement a previously reported method that quantified "inter"-muscular adipose tissue [23]. This method was further pre-clinically validated with animal experimentation by in vivo micro-CT and histological analysis.

2. Materials and Methods

2.1. Animal Grouping

In order to study intramuscular fat infiltration, it would be best to use a sarcopenia animal such as the senescence-accelerated mouse prone-8 (SAMP8) [5,24,25] with a documented intramuscular fat infiltration problem. However, limited by the small size of skeletal muscles on the SAMP8 mice for the HR-pQCT regarding measurements with sufficient resolution, the animal model selected was an ovariectomized Sprague Dawley (SD) rat model as estrogen deficiency was known to elevate adipogenesis and fat content in skeletal muscles [26,27]. Approval was granted from the Animal Experimentation Ethics Committee (AEEC) of the Chinese University of Hong Kong (CUHK) (Ref: 15-158-MIS).

Animals were fed with standard rat chow and allowed free cage movement. Bilateral ovariectomy or Sham operation was performed as previously described to 6-month-old SD rats and aged for 3 additional months according to our previous protocol [28,29]. After euthanasia with an overdose of 20% pentobarbital, muscle specimens were collected from 9-month-old ovariectomized (OVX, n = 4) and Sham-operated (SHAM, n = 4) female SD rats. Sample size was estimated based on the observed difference in intramuscular fat between normal and OVX rats of 30% and a SD of 15%, with a statistical power of 80% at an α level of 5%. The gastrocnemius in the lower leg of each rat was harvested for micro-CT and histological assessments.

2.2. Micro-CT Analysis of Animal Muscle

The specimens were scanned at a resolution of 8.4 µm isotropic voxel size at a beam energy of 70 kVp, current of 114 µA, and 200 ms of integration time (µCT40, Scanco Medical, Brüttisellen, Switzerland). A stack of sixty slices covering 0.480 mm were scanned at the middle of each gastrocnemius muscle. The images were analyzed using the manufacturer's evaluation program (µCT Evaluation Program v6.0, Scanco) according to a custom analysis protocol, determining the IMAT volume based on segmentation. Analyses of muscle tissues and IMAT were performed at the region of interest (ROI) consisting of a contour covering each muscle, spanning all slices of the scan. A Gaussian filter was applied to all images to reduce noise (sigma = 2.5, support = 5) as noise is known to influence the quantification of IMAT [30]. "Intra"-muscular IMAT was segmented using a lower threshold of −600 HU (Hounsfield units), which was supported by Erlandson et al. for the segmentation of fat for the evaluation of muscle and myotendinous tissue [23], and an upper threshold of 100 HU, which produced the best correlation between MD and IMAT in our preliminary study. To avoid border artefacts, the defined ROI was peeled with 3 voxels. The ROI, MD, and percentage of IMAT volume over the total ROI volume (IMAT%) were determined.

2.3. Histological Analysis of Animal Muscle

After micro-CT scanning, the muscle specimens were snap-frozen until cryo-sectioning. Muscle specimens were thawed and allowed to stabilize to the temperature of the microtome (CryoStar NX70, Thermo Fisher Scientific, Waltham, MA, USA) for 20 min. Muscle specimens were fixed with an OCT embedding compound (Tissue Tek, Sakura Finetek, CA, USA) and sectioned at 8 µm, and then thaw-mounted on silane-coated glass slides. Sections were then subject to hematoxylin and eosin (H&E) staining and oil red O (ORO) staining for the evaluation of intramuscular fat infiltration as previously described [5,31]. Briefly, for ORO staining, the slides were fixed in 10% formalin and 100% propylene glycol was added after incubation and washing. The slides were then stained with ORO solution for 10 min, counterstained with hematoxylin, and mounted with glycerin jelly mounting medium. Images were acquired using a light microscope (Leica DM5500 B, Leica Microsystems GmbH, Wetzlar, Germany) at 20× magnification. For each specimen, four images were analyzed by manually selecting the space between the cells containing connective and adipose tissue using graphical software (Adobe Photoshop CS6, Adobe Systems Inc., San José, CA, USA). Positive-stained areas were then quantified by color threshold using ImageJ software (version 1.52a, Wayne Rasband National Institutes of Health, Bethesda, Maryland, USA). The same thresholding values were used for all images in the semi-quantitative evaluation with hue: 228–255, saturation: 167–255, and brightness: 0–255. The stained area was expressed as the percentage (%) area fraction averaged from four separate images.

2.4. Subject Recruitment

Thirty adult Chinese female subjects from 18 to 81 years old (mean = 47.3 ± 19.2 years old) who suffered from a long bone fracture (femoral or tibial shaft) were recruited at the outpatient clinic of the Prince of Wales Hospital, Shatin, Hong Kong. Subjects were requested to take the HR-pQCT measurements, and muscle and functional assessments as described below. All assessments were performed in the Bone Quality and Health

Assessment Centre, Department of Orthopaedics and Traumatology, the Chinese University of Hong Kong, which is ISO 9001-certified for daily operation. The study protocol was approved by the Joint Chinese University of Hong Kong-New Territories East Cluster Clinical Research Ethics Committee (CRE-2008.530). Written informed consents were obtained from all subjects.

2.5. HR-pQCT Measurement of Subjects

The nonfractured-side distal tibias of all subjects were scanned by HR-pQCT (XtremeCT version I, Scanco Medical AG, Brüttisellen, Switzerland) using the standard patient protocol with an isotropic voxel size of 82 μm as our previous protocol [20]. The subject's leg was immobilized in a carbon fiber cast fixed within the scanner gantry. Proper positioning was ensured to minimize motion artefacts during scanning. A 2D scout view of the distal tibia was used to define the ROI. A reference line was placed at the end plate of the tibia. Measurements of 110 slices were acquired 22.5 mm proximal to the reference line. Each scan was carefully examined by the operator for motion artefacts, and up to two repeated scans at each site were performed in the case of significant motion artefacts. All images were graded for motion artefacts according to a visual grading system [32]. The short-term reproducibility of the vBMD parameter, expressed as the coefficient of variance, ranges from 0.38% to 1.03%, and the short-term reproducibility of microarchitectural parameters ranges from 0.80% to 3.73% [20,33].

2.6. Evaluation of Soft Tissue and Intramuscular Fat Content by HR-pQCT

The images were analyzed using the manufacturer's evaluation program (μCT Evaluation Program v6.0, Scanco) according to the Soft Tissue Analysis (STA) protocol (version 2.0) for the determination of the muscle ROI based on an earlier version of the STA protocol (version 1.0), previously described by Erlandson et al. to evaluate lean muscle and myotendinous tissue [23]. The method, however, only detects large areas of muscle and adipose tissue, leaving the IMAT undetected. In our modified protocol, we applied the STA protocol to optimize the thresholding method to isolate the muscle as the ROI for the segmentation and separation of lean and fat tissue within the muscle group for "intra"-muscular evaluation. Briefly, images were downscaled to 164 μm to reduce noise, followed by the exclusion of bone and skin from the analysis. The muscle and adipose tissues were defined by an iterative program using carefully adjusted thresholds to plant seed volumes in the soft tissues. By region growing, the soft tissue regions were defined after 20 iterations. The algorithm generated the contours of the muscle and adipose tissues and evaluated the total muscle volume (MV) in mm^3 and muscle density (MD) derived from the average attenuation coefficients in $mgHA/mm^3$ or HU. The default thresholds used were recommended by the manufacturer, 100 to 600 HU for muscle and -600 to -200 HU for fat (Figure 1). In our modified protocol, the threshold used for the segmentation of the IMAT was manually adjusted to -20 to 100 HU, as this threshold gave the most realistic results based on visual inspection (Figure 1). The settings for the Gaussian filters (sigma = 2.5, support = 5) remained unchanged.

2.7. Muscle Strength and Functional Assessment

The quadriceps and hamstring muscle strength on the nonfracture side were measured by instructing the subjects to perform an active extension of the knee joint in a sitting position with both feet free from the ground, and the hip and knee joint flexed at 90°. The peak isometric forces of the knee extension were measured by a dynamometer attached at the malleoli level. Measurements were repeated thrice and the maximum force was used for analysis as our previous protocol [34]. A chair rising test (CRT) was taken by each subject on the well-reported force plates (Leonardo Mechanograph, Novotec Medical, Pforzheim, Germany). Briefly, each subject was instructed to stand up until the knees were straight and immediately sat down for five consecutive times. Measurements were recorded by the built-in software and potential associations with HR-pQCT measurements were evaluated.

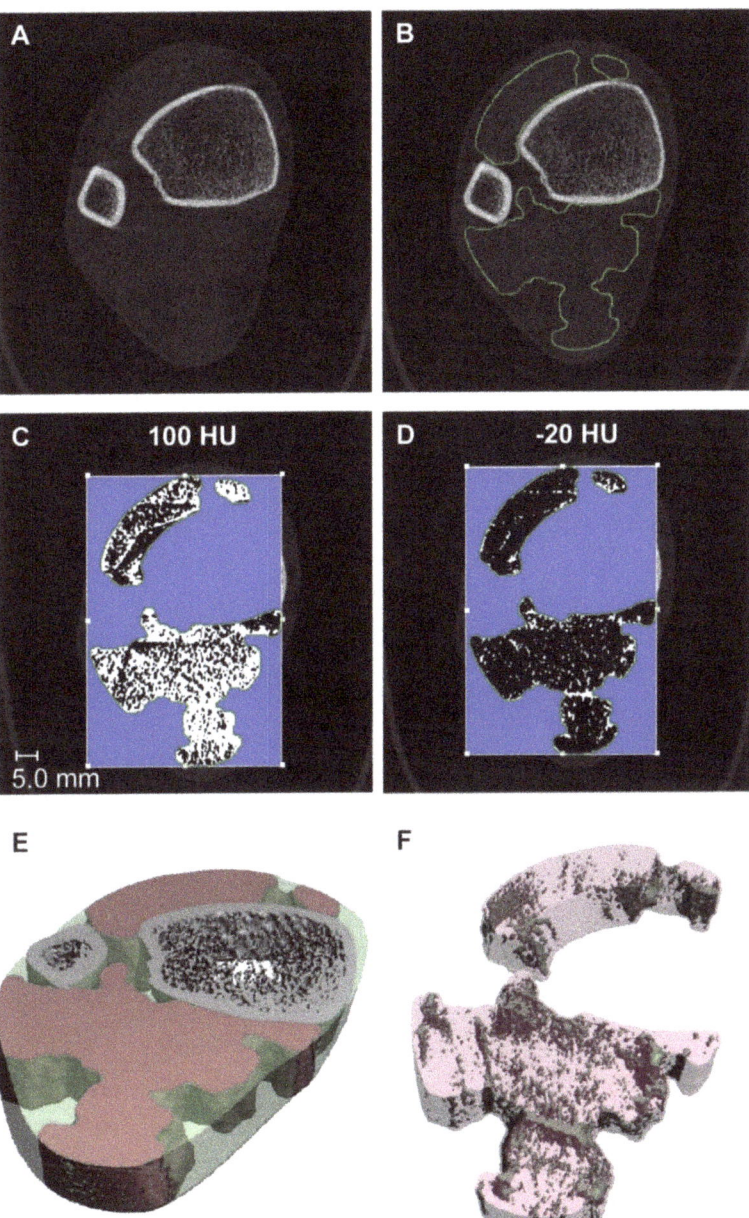

Figure 1. Representative images showing representation of the IMAT analysis protocol and the resulting 3D images. (**A**) In the original image, the ROI was selected using the muscle contours determined by the STA protocol, which is (**B**) depicted in green. (**C**) The intended segmentation threshold with an upper threshold of 100 HU did not produce a realistic result and was, therefore, rejected. (**D**) The upper threshold of −20 HU was defined manually. (**E**) The STA protocol produces a 3D segmentation, with the bones depicted in grey, the muscles in red, and fat in transparent green. (**F**) Application of the IMAT segmentation produces a 3D image, as shown with the IMAT depicted in green and the muscle depicted in transparent red.

2.8. Statistical Analysis

An independent Student's *t*-test was conducted to analyze the data of the SHAM and OVX rats. The potential association between IMAT%, MD, and ORO area was evaluated with Pearson's correlations. For the clinical part, linear regression analysis was performed and the coefficient of determination (R^2) was calculated to analyze the relationship between age and MD, and between age and the amount of IMAT in the defined muscle regions. The Pearson correlation coefficient (r) was calculated to determine the degree of correlation between the IMAT, MD, and chair rise time. All statistical analyses were performed using Prism (version 6.01, GraphPad Software, Inc., San Diego, CA, USA). $p < 0.05$ was regarded as statistically significant, and the Shapiro–Wilk normality test was used where necessary.

3. Results

3.1. IMAT and MD Reflect Intramuscular Fat Content and Muscle Quality in Rats

Micro-CT results showed that IMAT% was significantly higher ($p = 0.03$) in OVX rats than in SHAM rats (Figure 2A). However, no significance was detected for MD between the two groups (Figure 2B). Histologically, from the H&E staining, the OVX group presented more intramuscular fat tissue than the SHAM group (Figure 3A). Oil red O staining was used to analyze the fat infiltration in skeletal muscle tissue of the SHAM and OVX rats. The OVX group showed a 160% higher ORO area compared to the SHAM group ($p = 0.03$) (Figure 3B,C). The IMAT% evaluated by the microCT was shown to be 39% higher in the OVX group, and was strongly associated with the ORO-positively stained area (r = 0.898, $p = 0.002$) (Figure 4).

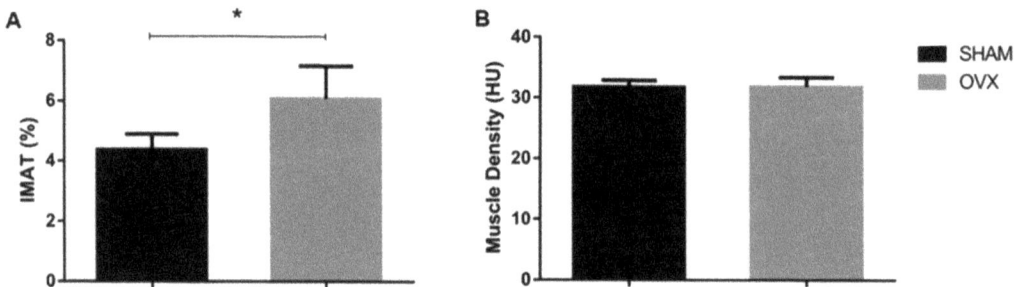

Figure 2. (**A**) IMAT% was significantly higher in OVX rats than in SHAM rats (* $p < 0.05$). (**B**) No significance was detected for MD between the two groups.

3.2. HR-pQCT Parameters Associated with Intramuscular Fat Content and Muscle Performance

Of the HR-pQCT parameters produced, a moderate positive correlation was detected between MV and MD (r = 0.642, $p < 0.001$), and between MV and IMAT volume (r = 0.618, $p < 0.01$). Moderate negative correlations were detected between MD and IMAT% (r = −0.640, $p < 0.001$).

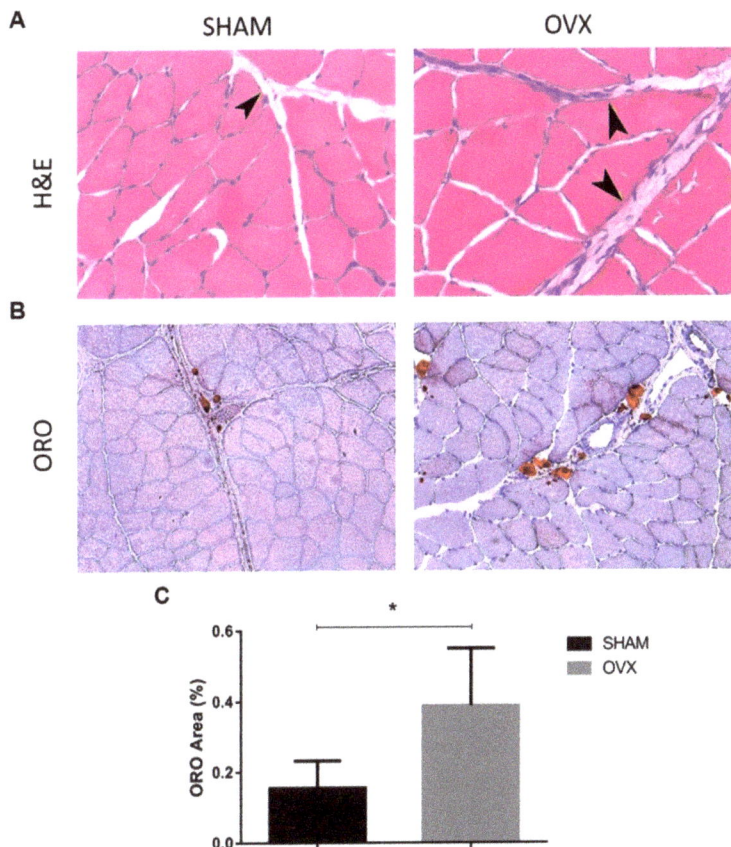

Figure 3. Morphological differences and fat infiltration of skeletal muscles in SHAM and OVX rats. (**A**) The OVX group presented more intramuscular fat tissue than the SHAM group by H&E taken at 20× magnification, where fat tissues are indicated by black arrows. (**B**) The OVX group showed a higher ORO signal (red area) than the SHAM group. (**C**) Quantitative analysis revealed that the ORO area of the OVX group was significantly higher (* $p < 0.05$, Student's T-test).

The age of the participants was found to be negatively associated with HR-pQCT parameters, including MV (r = −0.479, $p < 0.01$), IMAT/MV (r = 0.620, $p < 0.01$), MD (r = −0.763, $p < 0.05$), and MCSA (r = −0.479, $p < 0.05$), and positively correlated with IMAT% (r = 0.559, $p < 0.01$), all with statistical significance (Table 1). Age was also found to correlate with all muscle strength and performance outcomes, with a moderate to strong correlation detected with Pmax (r = −0.608, $p < 0.001$) of the chair rise test, and both the quadriceps and hamstring strength (r = −0.686 and r = −0.638, respectively, both at $p < 0.01$, Table 2).

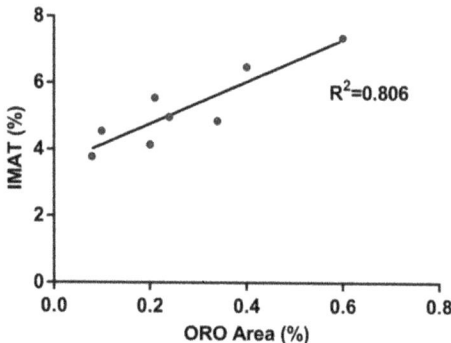

Figure 4. MicroCT fat-related parameter of IMAT% was highly correlated with ORO-positively stained area (r = 0.898, r^2 = 0.806; $p < 0.05$).

Table 1. Correlations between age and various muscle-related parameters produced by HR-pQCT.

	Tibia CSA [cm²]	Total.Volume	Muscle.Volume	MV/TV	IMAT.Volume	IMAT/MV	Muscle.Density	Fat.Density	MCSA	IMAT.V	MUS.V	IMAT%
Age	−0.504	−0.380	−0.479 *	−0.208	0.309	0.620 **	−0.763 **	−0.074	−0.479 *	0.070	−0.483 *	0.559 **

Significant correlations were found in MV, IMAT/MV, MD, and IMAT%. * and ** represent significant correlations at the 0.05 and 0.01 levels (2-tailed), respectively.

Table 2. Correlations between various muscle-related parameters produced by HR-pQCT and functional parameters of the subjects.

	P_{max}	P_{max} (Fracture)	P_{max} ((Normal))	Total Time	Time per Test	Rise Time	Quadriceps Strength	Hamstring Strength
Age	−0.608 **	−0.406	−0.633 **	0.507 *	0.514 *	0.434 *	−0.686 **	−0.638 **
Tibia CSA	0.615 *	0.313	0.653 *	−0.112	−0.304	−0.099	0.468	0.454
TV	0.631 **	0.497 *	0.619 **	−0.104	−0.306	−0.085	0.438 *	0.330
MV	0.317	0.207	0.338	−0.413 *	−0.354	−0.476 *	0.245	0.282
MV/TV	−0.236	−0.203	−0.219	−0.377	−0.097	−0.441 *	−0.078	0.064
IMAT.V.	−0.070	0.002	−0.095	0.211	0.112	0.168	−0.385	−0.279
IMAT/MV	−0.214	−0.089	−0.249	0.452 *	0.298	0.525 *	−0.560 **	−0.429 *
MD	0.444 *	0.262	0.489 *	−0.704 **	−0.625 **	−0.610 **	0.588 **	0.565 **
FD	−0.306	−0.296	−0.267	−0.192	0.152	−0.156	−0.213	−0.024
MCSA	0.317	0.207	0.338	−0.413 *	−0.354	−0.476 *	0.245	0.282
• IMAT.V	0.003	−0.067	0.052	0.055	0.024	0.086	−0.273	−0.080
• MUS.V	0.301	0.190	0.327	−0.486 *	−0.384	−0.515 *	0.254	0.291
• IMAT%	−0.245	−0.252	−0.200	0.436 *	0.311	0.671 **	−0.559 **	−0.380

Muscle Density (MD) and IMAT% were found to be the most predictive parameters with statistically significant correlations. * and ** represent significant correlations at the 0.05 and 0.01 levels (2-tailed), respectively. Abbreviations: CSA = cross-sectional area, TV = tissue volume, MV = muscle volume, D = density, AT = adipose tissue. • Designates measurements from the modified protocol.

HR-pQCT-evaluated soft tissue parameters were found to associate moderately with functional outcomes including TV vs. P_{max} (r = 0.631, $p < 0.01$), MD vs. P_{max} (r = 0.444, $p < 0.05$), MD vs. quadriceps strength (r = 0.588, $p < 0.01$), and MD vs. hamstring strength (r = 0.565). Furthermore, the fat-related parameter of IMAT% was found to be statistically associated with rise time (r = 0.671, $p < 0.01$) and quadriceps strength (r = -0.559, $p < 0.001$), all with statistical significances (Table 2).

4. Discussion

The current study attempted to verify and provide scientific evidence to support the utilization of HR-pQCT for the evaluation of muscle quality and the detection of intramuscular fat infiltration, which is potentially applicable for the diagnosis or identification of sarcopenia for personalized intervention decisions. It is highly clinically significant for the prevention of falls and fragility fractures during musculoskeletal ageing. From the results of evaluating animal samples and human scans, CT parameters correlated well with the intramuscular fat content and muscle performance. Our results showed that HR-pQCT not only has the advantage of providing added structural information of bone tissue over the course of the ageing process [20], but also the capability of evaluating the quality of muscle down to the smallest changes in muscle density and predicting intramuscular fat infiltration. Therefore, it is a feasible method to be utilized clinically for bone and muscle evaluation with just a single scan.

The initial aim of the pre-clinical study was to implement the IMAT protocol using the upper threshold with the best results. However, the IMAT segmentation using this threshold (100 HU) resulted in unrealistic results, as shown in Figure 1C. This was most likely due to the lower resolution of the HR-pQCT (82 µm) compared to the µCT images of the rat leg (8.4 µm), causing high interference of partial volumes. Additionally, the human images were made with a different scanner, which could influence the linear attenuation measured. Therefore, a new upper threshold of -20 HU was determined visually, which resulted in a strong correlation with the measured MD. Nevertheless, the accuracy of this threshold remains subjective, as is shown by the discrepancy of the segmented adipose tissue area (39% higher in OVX) and the histological lipid deposition area (160% higher in the OVX), indicating an underestimated intramuscular fat content by the microCT; therefore, it should be further validated. A similar validation study performed in the pre-clinical study could also be performed on human subjects, but retrieving muscle biopsies from patients can be challenging. An alternative could be post-mortem studies, although muscle tissue quickly deteriorates after death.

Myosteatosis, or intramuscular fat infiltration, has attracted increasing attention recently due to the escalating aging population, and it is recognized as one of the many causes of sarcopenia. Many factors may cause this to happen during the aging process, including a lack of physical activities or mechanical stimulation [35], changes in the adipogenic or myogenic properties of muscle stem cells [5], and estrogen deficiency [36]. Muscle quantification and evaluation can be performed with various imaging modalities including magnetic resonance imaging (MRI), dual-energy X-ray absorptiometry (DXA), and peripheral quantitative computed tomography (pQCT), each with their pros, cons, and limitations of accessibility [37]. Until a further consensus of standardized protocol by MRI or another imaging protocol is reached for the evaluation of intermuscular or intramuscular fatty content [17], HR-pQCT could be one possible alternative that has the advantage of producing high-resolution bone, muscle, and adipose tissue data with a very low radiation dosage (~3 µSv per scan) that can be performed relatively quickly [38]. However, little research has been conducted to evaluate its use in skeletal muscle. Erlandson et al. compared the muscle-related parameters produced by the HR-pQCT against the more conventional pQCT and found that both muscle density and cross-sectional areas correlated well [23,39], and they suggested that the HR-pQCT can be used to evaluate the amount of myotendinous tissue (Mt) and quantification of muscle density (MD). Their conclusion is also supported by our current study, indicating that the HR-pQCT parameters of the muscle density (MD) and intramuscular IMAT% correlated well with age and muscle functions. Recently, Hildebrand et al. also demonstrated good precision and repeatability of the HR-pQCT against the more traditional method of pQCT that also supports its potential clinical application [40]. Furthermore, this is supported with our animal study showing that the IMAT% evaluated by the HR-pQCT had a moderately strong correlation ($r^2 = 0.806$) with the quantification of intramuscular lipids by Oil Red O histology. Although HR-pQCT is disadvantageous to MRI, limited to its ability to differentiate various soft tissues [23], from our findings in this study, we recommend the use of this imaging modality as a rapid evaluation of muscle quality and objective quantification of skeletal muscle at the peripheral for sarcopenia assessment, while gathering bone micro-architectural parameters is important for osteoporosis and fracture risk prediction [41] in order to tackle two disease in one go for the prevention of fragility fracture.

The chair rise time has been shown to be a good predictive tool for sarcopenia in elderly women by Pinheiro et al. [42]. Additionally, Patel et al. [43] showed that women without sarcopenia completed the chair rise test faster than women with sarcopenia. The results from this study showed a moderate positive relationship between the chair rise time and IMAT, suggesting that the IMAT content is higher in patients with a longer chair rise time. It should be noted that the studies by Pinheiro et al. and Patel et al. only included elderly participants, while this study included young and elderly patients. Therefore, IMAT content is predictive of physical performance during the age-related changes in skeletal muscles.

The literature has shown that an increase in IMAT is not only related to sarcopenia [14] but also to an increase in BMI in both young and elderly populations [44]. Any changes in MD, IMAT, and chair rise time in this study can be related to either age, BMI, or a combination of these two factors. One limitation of our study is that anthropometric measures of fractured subjects were not collected nor taken into account. Nevertheless, as this was a study to investigate the potential of the IMAT protocol on HR-pQCT as an imaging modality, these factors did not have a major impairment to the success of this study.

5. Conclusions

The modified HR-pQCT evaluation protocol produced MD and IMAT results that were associated with age and physical performance measures and were of good predictive value for the progression of myosteatosis. The protocol was validated on animal skeletal muscle samples that further support the clinical application for the rapid evaluation of muscle quality and the objective quantification of skeletal muscle at the peripheral for sarcopenia assessment.

Author Contributions: Conceptualization, S.K.-H.C., R.M.-Y.W., K.-S.L., and W.-H.C.; methodology, S.K.-H.C., M.v.M., N.Z., V.W.-Y.H., and M.M.-C.L..; software, M.v.M.; data analysis, M.v.M., M.M.-C.L., N.Z.; writing—original draft preparation, M.v.M. and S.K.-H.C.; writing—review and editing, M.v.M., S.K.-H.C., and W.-H.C.; visualization, M.v.M. and S.K.-H.C.; supervision, R.M.-Y.W., K.-S.L., and W.-H.C.; project administration, S.K.-H.C. and W.-H.C.; funding acquisition, K.-S.L., R.M.-Y.W., S.K.-H.C., and W.-H.C. All authors have read and agreed to the published version of the manuscript.

Funding: The research was partly supported by the Healthcare and Promotion Scheme (HCPS, Ref: 02180118), HMRF-Research Fellowship Scheme (Ref: 06200037), and the RGC-CRF (Ref: C4032-21GF).

Institutional Review Board Statement: The study protocol involving animal specimens was granted approval from the Animal Experimentation Ethics Committee (AEEC) of the Chinese University of Hong Kong (CUHK) (Ref: 15-158-MIS). The study protocol involving human subjects was approved by the Joint Chinese University of Hong Kong-New Territories East Cluster Clinical Research Ethics Committee (CRE-2008.530).

Informed Consent Statement: Informed consent was obtained from all subjects involved in the study.

Data Availability Statement: The data presented in this study are available on request from the corresponding author. The data are not publicly available, due to restrictions from institutional ethics approval.

Acknowledgments: The authors would like to thank the support of Chim Yu Ning, Keith Cheng, and Valerie Li for their histology work and Habiba Akter for research administrative support.

Conflicts of Interest: The authors declare no conflict of interest.

References

1. Cruz-Jentoft, A.J.; Sayer, A.A. Sarcopenia. *Lancet* **2019**, *393*, 2636–2646. [CrossRef]
2. Wong, R.M.Y.; Wong, H.; Zhang, N.; Chow, S.K.H.; Chau, W.W.; Wang, J.; Chim, Y.N.; Leung, K.S.; Cheung, W.H. The relationship between sarcopenia and fragility fracture-a systematic review. *Osteoporos. Int.* **2019**, *30*, 541–553. [CrossRef] [PubMed]
3. Health AgingBody Composition Study; Delmonico, M.J.; Harris, T.B.; Visser, M.; Park, S.W.; Conroy, M.B.; Velasquez-Mieyer, P.; Boudreau, R.; Manini, T.M.; Nevitt, M.; et al. Longitudinal study of muscle strength, quality, and adipose tissue infiltration. *Am. J. Clin. Nutr.* **2009**, *90*, 1579–1585. [CrossRef]
4. Goodpaster, B.H.; Carlson, C.L.; Visser, M.; Kelley, D.E.; Scherzinger, A.; Harris, T.B.; Stamm, E.; Newman, A.B. Attenuation of skeletal muscle and strength in the elderly: The Health ABC Study. *J. Appl. Physiol.* **2001**, *90*, 2157–2165. [CrossRef] [PubMed]
5. Wang, J.; Cui, C.; Chim, Y.N.; Yao, H.; Shi, L.; Xu, J.; Wang, J.; Wong, R.M.Y.; Leung, K.; Chow, S.K.; et al. Vibration and beta-hydroxy-beta-methylbutyrate treatment suppresses intramuscular fat infiltration and adipogenic differentiation in sarcopenic mice. *J. Cachexia Sarcopenia Muscle* **2020**, *11*, 564–577. [CrossRef]
6. Cruz-Jentoft, A.J.; Baeyens, J.P.; Bauer, J.M.; Boirie, Y.; Cederholm, T.; Landi, F.; Martin, F.C.; Michel, J.-P.; Rolland, Y.; Schneider, S.M.; et al. Sarcopenia: European consensus on definition and diagnosis: Report of the European Working Group on Sarcopenia in Older People. *Age Ageing* **2010**, *39*, 412–423. [CrossRef]
7. Cruz-Jentoft, A.J.; Bahat, G.; Bauer, J.; Boirie, Y.; Bruyère, O.; Cederholm, T.; Cooper, C.; Landi, F.; Rolland, Y.; Sayer, A.A.; et al. Sarcopenia: Revised European consensus on definition and diagnosis. *Age Ageing* **2019**, *48*, 16–31. [CrossRef]
8. Chen, L.K.; Liu, L.-K.; Woo, J.; Assantachai, P.; Auyeung, T.-W.; Bahyah, K.S.; Chou, M.-Y.; Chen, L.-Y.; Hsu, P.-S.; Krairit, O.; et al. Sarcopenia in Asia: Consensus report of the Asian Working Group for Sarcopenia. *J. Am. Med. Dir. Assoc.* **2014**, *15*, 95–101. [CrossRef]
9. Shafiee, G.; Keshtkar, A.; Soltani, A.; Ahadi, Z.; Larijani, B.; Heshmat, R. Prevalence of sarcopenia in the world: A systematic review and meta- analysis of general population studies. *J. Diabetes Metab. Disord.* **2017**, *16*, 21. [CrossRef]
10. Scott, D.; Seibel, M.; Cumming, R.; Naganathan, V.; Blyth, F.; Le Couteur, D.; Handelsman, D.J.; Waite, L.M.; Hirani, V. Sarcopenic Obesity and Its Temporal Associations With Changes in Bone Mineral Density, Incident Falls, and Fractures in Older Men: The Concord Health and Ageing in Men Project. *J. Bone Miner. Res. Off. J. Am. Soc. Bone Miner. Res.* **2017**, *32*, 575–583. [CrossRef]
11. Yu, R.; Leung, J.; Woo, J. Incremental predictive value of sarcopenia for incident fracture in an elderly Chinese cohort: Results from the Osteoporotic Fractures in Men (MrOs) Study. *J. Am. Med. Dir. Assoc.* **2014**, *15*, 551–558. [CrossRef] [PubMed]
12. Heymsfield, S.B.; Adamek, M.; Gonzalez, M.C.; Jia, G.; Thomas, D.M. Assessing skeletal muscle mass: Historical overview and state of the art. *J. Cachexia Sarcopenia Muscle* **2014**, *5*, 9–18. [CrossRef] [PubMed]
13. Ogawa, M.; Lester, R.; Akima, H.; Gorgey, A.S. Quantification of intermuscular and intramuscular adipose tissue using magnetic resonance imaging after neurodegenerative disorders. *Neural Regen. Res.* **2017**, *12*, 2100–2105. [CrossRef] [PubMed]
14. Marcus, R.L.; Addison, O.; Dibble, L.E.; Foreman, K.B.; Morrell, G.; LaStayo, P. Intramuscular adipose tissue, sarcopenia, and mobility function in older individuals. *J. Aging Res.* **2012**, *2012*, 629637. [CrossRef] [PubMed]
15. Maddocks, M.; Shrikrishna, D.; Vitoriano, S.; Natanek, S.A.; Tanner, R.J.; Hart, N.; Kemp, P.R.; Moxham, J.; Polkey, M.I.; Hopkinson, N.S. Skeletal muscle adiposity is associated with physical activity, exercise capacity and fibre shift in COPD. *Eur. Respir. J.* **2014**, *44*, 1188–1198. [CrossRef]
16. Borkan, G.A.; Hults, D.E.; Gerzof, S.G.; Robbins, A.H.; Silbert, C.K. Age changes in body composition revealed by computed tomography. *J. Gerontol.* **1983**, *38*, 673–677. [CrossRef]
17. Wong, A.K.O.; Szabo, E.; Erlandson, M.; Sussman, M.S.; Duggina, S.; Song, A.; Reitsma, S.; Gillick, H.; Adachi, J.D.; Cheung, A.M. A Valid and Precise Semiautomated Method for Quantifying INTERmuscular Fat INTRAmuscular Fat in Lower Leg Magnetic Resonance Images. *J. Clin. Densitom.* **2018**, *23*, 611–622. [CrossRef]
18. Sunil, K.C. Hong Kong Free Press: Years-long waiting times at Hong Kong hospitals – inefficient at best, corrupt at wors. Hong Kong. 2018. Available online: https://hongkongfp.com/2018/12/30/years-long-waiting-times-hong-kong-hospitals-inefficient-best-corrupt-worse/ (accessed on 21 June 2021).
19. Cheng, K.Y.; Chow, S.K.; Hung, V.W.; Wong, C.H.; Wong, R.M.; Tsang, C.S.; Kwok, T.; Cheung, W. Diagnosis of sarcopenia by evaluating skeletal muscle mass by adjusted bioimpedance analysis validated with dual-energy X-ray absorptiometry. *J. Cachexia Sarcopenia Muscle* **2021**, *12*, 2163–2173. [CrossRef]
20. Hung, V.W.; Zhu, T.; Cheung, W.H.; Fong, T.-N.; Yu, F.W.P.; Hung, L.-K.; Leung, K.-S.; Cheng, J.; Lam, T.-P.; Qin, L. Age-related differences in volumetric bone mineral density, microarchitecture, and bone strength of distal radius and tibia in Chinese women: A high-resolution pQCT reference database study. *Osteoporos. Int.* **2015**, *26*, 1691–1703. [CrossRef]

21. Zhu, T.Y.; Hung, V.W.Y.; Cheung, W.-H.; Cheng, J.C.Y.; Qin, L.; Leung, K.-S. Value of Measuring Bone Microarchitecture in Fracture Discrimination in Older Women with Recent Hip Fracture: A Case-control Study with HR-pQCT. *Sci. Rep.* **2016**, *6*, 34185. [CrossRef]
22. Cheung, W.H.; Hung, V.W.; Cheuk, K.; Chau, W.; Tsoi, K.K.; Wong, R.M.; Chow, S.K.; Lam, T.; Yung, P.S.; Law, S.; et al. Best Performance Parameters of HR-pQCT to Predict Fragility Fracture: Systematic Review and Meta-Analysis. *J. Bone Miner. Res. Off. J. Am. Soc. Bone Miner. Res.* **2021**, *36*, 2381–2398. [CrossRef] [PubMed]
23. Erlandson, M.C.; Wong, A.; Szabo, E.; Vilayphiou, N.; Zulliger, M.; Adachi, J.; Cheung, A. Muscle and Myotendinous Tissue Properties at the Distal Tibia as Assessed by High-Resolution Peripheral Quantitative Computed Tomography. *J. Clin. Densitom.* **2017**, *20*, 226–232. [CrossRef] [PubMed]
24. Guo, A.Y.; Leung, K.S.; Qin, J.H.; Chow, S.K.; Cheung, W.H. Effect of Low-Magnitude, High-Frequency Vibration Treatment on Retardation of Sarcopenia: Senescence-Accelerated Mouse-P8 Model. *Rejuvenation Res.* **2016**, *19*, 293–302. [CrossRef] [PubMed]
25. Guo, A.Y.; Leung, K.S.; Siu, P.M.F.; Qin, J.H.; Chow, S.K.H.; Qin, L.; Li, C.Y.; Cheung, W.H. Muscle mass, structural and functional investigations of senescence-accelerated mouse P8 (SAMP8). *Exp. Anim.* **2015**, *64*, 425–433. [CrossRef] [PubMed]
26. Frechette, D.M.; Krishnamoorthy, D.; Adler, B.J.; Chan, M.E.; Rubin, C.T. Diminished satellite cells and elevated adipogenic gene expression in muscle as caused by ovariectomy are averted by low-magnitude mechanical signals. *J. Appl. Physiol.* **2015**, *119*, 27–36. [CrossRef]
27. Leite, R.D.; Prestes, J.; Bernardes, C.F.; Shiguemoto, G.E.; Pereira, G.B.; Duarte, J.O.; Domingos, M.M.; Baldissera, V.; Perez, S.E.D.A. Effects of ovariectomy and resistance training on lipid content in skeletal muscle, liver, and heart; fat depots; and lipid profile. *Appl. Physiol. Nutr. Metab. Physiol. Appl. Nutr. Metab.* **2009**, *34*, 1079–1086. [CrossRef]
28. Chow, S.K.; Leung, K.S.; Qin, J.; Guo, A.; Sun, M.; Qin, L.; Cheung, W.H. Mechanical stimulation enhanced estrogen receptor expression and callus formation in diaphyseal long bone fracture healing in ovariectomy-induced osteoporotic rats. *Osteoporos. Int.* **2016**, *27*, 2989–3000. [CrossRef]
29. Shi, H.F.; Cheung, W.H.; Qin, L.; Leung, A.H.; Leung, K.S. Low-magnitude high-frequency vibration treatment augments fracture healing in ovariectomy-induced osteoporotic bone. *Bone* **2010**, *46*, 1299–1305. [CrossRef] [PubMed]
30. Butner, K.L.; Creamer, K.W.; Nickols-Richardson, S.M.; Clark, S.F.; Ramp, W.K.; Herbert, W.G. Fat and muscle indices assessed by pQCT: Relationships with physical activity and type 2 diabetes risk. *J. Clin. Densitom.* **2012**, *15*, 355–361. [CrossRef] [PubMed]
31. Mehlem, A.; Hagberg, C.E.; Muhl, L.; Eriksson, U.; Falkevall, A. Imaging of neutral lipids by oil red O for analyzing the metabolic status in health and disease. *Nat. Protoc.* **2013**, *8*, 1149–1154. [CrossRef]
32. Engelke, K.; Stampa, B.; Timm, W.; Dardzinski, B.; de Papp, A.E.; Genant, H.K.; Fuerst, T. Short-term in vivo precision of BMD and parameters of trabecular architecture at the distal forearm and tibia. *Osteoporos. Int.* **2012**, *23*, 2151–2158. [CrossRef] [PubMed]
33. Zhu, T.Y.; Yip, B.H.; Hung, V.W.; Choy, C.W.; Cheng, K.-L.; Kwok, T.C.; Cheng, J.; Qin, L. Normative Standards for HRpQCT Parameters in Chinese Men and Women. *J. Bone Miner. Res. Off. J. Am. Soc. Bone Miner. Res.* **2018**, *33*, 1889–1899. [CrossRef]
34. Leung, K.S.; Li, C.Y.; Tse, Y.K.; Choy, T.K.; Leung, P.C.; Hung, V.W.Y.; Chan, S.Y.; Leung, A.H.C.; Cheung, W.H. Effects of 18-month low-magnitude high-frequency vibration on fall rate and fracture risks in 710 community elderly—A cluster-randomized controlled trial. *Osteoporos. Int.* **2014**, *25*, 1785–1795. [CrossRef] [PubMed]
35. Rubin, C.T.; Capilla, E.; Luu, Y.K.; Busa, B.; Crawford, H.; Nolan, D.J.; Mittal, V.; Rosen, C.J.; Pessin, J.E.; Judex, S. Adipogenesis is inhibited by brief, daily exposure to high-frequency, extremely low-magnitude mechanical signals. *Proc. Natl. Acad. Sci. USA* **2007**, *104*, 17879–17884. [CrossRef] [PubMed]
36. Hamrick, M.W.; McGee-Lawrence, M.E.; Frechette, D.M. Fatty Infiltration of Skeletal Muscle: Mechanisms and Comparisons with Bone Marrow Adiposity. *Front. Endocrinol.* **2016**, *7*, 69. [CrossRef]
37. Wong, A.K. A comparison of peripheral imaging technologies for bone and muscle quantification: A technical review of image acquisition. *J. Musculoskelet. Neuronal Interact.* **2016**, *16*, 265–282.
38. Nishiyama, K.K.; Shane, E. Clinical imaging of bone microarchitecture with HR-pQCT. *Curr. Osteoporos. Rep.* **2013**, *11*, 147–155. [CrossRef]
39. Erlandson, M.C.; Lorbergs, A.L.; Mathur, S.; Cheung, A.M. Muscle analysis using pQCT, DXA and MRI. *Eur. J. Radiol.* **2016**, *85*, 1505–1511. [CrossRef]
40. Hildebrand, K.N.; Sidhu, K.; Gabel, L.; Besler, B.A.; Burt, L.A.; Boyd, S.K. The Assessment of Skeletal Muscle and Cortical Bone by Second-generation HR-pQCT at the Tibial Midshaft. *J. Clin. Densitom.* **2021**, *24*, 465–473. [CrossRef]
41. Samelson, E.J.; Broe, K.E.; Xu, H.; Yang, L.; Boyd, S.; Biver, E.; Szulc, P.; Adachi, J.; Amin, S.; Atkinson, E.; et al. Cortical and trabecular bone microarchitecture as an independent predictor of incident fracture risk in older women and men in the Bone Microarchitecture International Consortium (BoMIC): A prospective study. *Lancet Diabetes Endocrinol.* **2019**, *7*, 34–43. [CrossRef]
42. Pinheiro, P.A.; Carneiro, J.A.; Coqueiro, R.S.; Pereira, R.; Fernandes, M.H. "Chair Stand Test" as Simple Tool for Sarcopenia Screening in Elderly Women. *J. Nutr. Health Aging* **2016**, *20*, 56–59. [CrossRef] [PubMed]
43. Patel, H.P.; Syddall, H.E.; Jameson, K.; Robinson, S.; Denison, H.; Roberts, H.C.; Edwards, M.; Dennison, E.; Cooper, C.; Aihie Sayer, A. Prevalence of sarcopenia in community-dwelling older people in the UK using the European Working Group on Sarcopenia in Older People (EWGSOP) definition: Findings from the Hertfordshire Cohort Study (HCS). *Age Ageing* **2013**, *42*, 378–384. [CrossRef] [PubMed]
44. Vettor, R.; Milan, G.; Franzin, C.; Sanna, M.; De Coppi, P.; Rizzuto, R.; Federspil, G. The origin of intermuscular adipose tissue and its pathophysiological implications. *Am. J. Physiol. Endocrinol. Metab.* **2009**, *297*, E987–E998. [CrossRef] [PubMed]

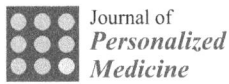

Article

Serum and Synovial Markers in Patients with Rheumatoid Arthritis and Periprosthetic Joint Infection

Yi Ren [1], Lara Biedermann [1], Clemens Gwinner [1], Carsten Perka [1] and Arne Kienzle [1,2,*]

[1] Center for Musculoskeletal Surgery, Clinic for Orthopedics, Charité University Hospital, 10117 Berlin, Germany; yi.ren@charite.de (Y.R.); lara.biedermann@charite.de (L.B.); clemens.gwinner@charite.de (C.G.); carsten.perka@charite.de (C.P.)
[2] Berlin Institute of Health, Charité—Universitätsmedizin Berlin, BIH Biomedical Innovation Academy, BIH Charité Clinician Scientist Program, Charitéplatz 1, 10117 Berlin, Germany
* Correspondence: arne.kienzle@charite.de; Tel.: +49-30-450-615739

Citation: Ren, Y.; Biedermann, L.; Gwinner, C.; Perka, C.; Kienzle, A. Serum and Synovial Markers in Patients with Rheumatoid Arthritis and Periprosthetic Joint Infection. *J. Pers. Med.* **2022**, *12*, 810. https://doi.org/10.3390/jpm12050810

Academic Editor: Dilia Giuggioli

Received: 8 April 2022
Accepted: 12 May 2022
Published: 17 May 2022

Publisher's Note: MDPI stays neutral with regard to jurisdictional claims in published maps and institutional affiliations.

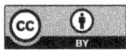

Copyright: © 2022 by the authors. Licensee MDPI, Basel, Switzerland. This article is an open access article distributed under the terms and conditions of the Creative Commons Attribution (CC BY) license (https://creativecommons.org/licenses/by/4.0/).

Abstract: Current diagnostic standards for PJI rely on inflammatory markers that are typically elevated in autoimmune diseases, thus making the diagnosis of PJI in patients with rheumatoid arthritis and joint replacement particularly complicated. There is a paucity of data on differentiating PJI from rheumatoid arthritis in patients with previous arthroplasty. In this study, we retrospectively analyzed the cases of 17 patients with rheumatoid arthritis and 121 patients without rheumatoid disease who underwent surgical intervention due to microbiology-positive PJI of the hip or knee joint. We assessed clinical patient characteristics, laboratory parameters, and prosthesis survival rates in patients with and without rheumatoid arthritis and acute or chronic PJI. ROC analysis was conducted for the analyzed parameters. In patients with chronic PJI, peripheral blood CRP ($p = 0.05$, AUC = 0.71), synovial WBC count ($p = 0.02$, AUC = 0.78), synovial monocyte cell count ($p = 0.04$, AUC = 0.75), and synovial PMN cell count ($p = 0.02$, AUC = 0.80) were significantly elevated in patients with rheumatoid arthritis showing acceptable to excellent discrimination. All analyzed parameters showed no significant differences and poor discrimination for patients with acute PJI. Median prosthesis survival time was significantly shorter in patients with rheumatoid arthritis ($p = 0.05$). In conclusion, routinely used laboratory markers have limited utility in distinguishing acute PJI in rheumatoid patients. In cases with suspected chronic PJI but low levels of serum CRP and synovial cell markers, physicians should consider the possibility of activated autoimmune arthritis.

Keywords: periprosthetic joint infection; rheumatoid arthritis; arthroplasty; total knee replacement; total hip replacement

1. Introduction

PJI is a major complication following joint replacement occurring in 1–5% of patients with primary arthroplasties [1,2]. Depending on the duration of symptoms, PJI is classified as acute or chronic. While the exact cutoff value is of ongoing debate, acute PJI is commonly defined as an infection with symptom duration ≤ 4 weeks [3,4]. In chronic PJI, symptoms have been present for > 4 weeks and may be the result of a low-virulence organism [5]. In both cases, adequate surgical treatment of PJI is mandatory to achieve a successful, infection-free outcome [6,7]. While treatment with debridement and implant retention can be an effective therapy for acute PJI, one- or two-stage exchange surgery may be required in chronic PJI [8]. In any of these cases, treatment is an enormous burden for patients [9]. In addition to surgical intervention, exchange arthroplasty can significantly impact joint function, cause pain, and has an increased risk of prosthesis failure [10–12].

Attending physicians are often challenged by the need to accurately diagnose PJI within a short time frame to be able to decide upon the necessary treatment strategy. Despite significant progress in recent years, no agreed-upon gold standard for the diagnosis of PJI exists [13]. Besides clinical presentation, diagnosis usually relies upon laboratory diagnostics using peripheral blood as well as synovial fluid. The markers routinely used are WBC count and serum CRP, as well as synovial WBC count and PMN cell percentage [14,15]. Depending on national, regional, or hospital-specific guidelines and standards, additional testing for leukocyte esterase, alpha-defensin, D-dimer, erythrocyte sedimentation rate, and synovial CRP may be performed. Additionally, microbiological culture is essential but not feasible in an acute setting due to culture time [16]. In some cases, microbiological culture may be negative despite the presence of PJI [17,18].

While both the 2018 Definition of Periprosthetic Hip and Knee Infection by Parvizi et al. and the EBJIS definition of PJI are reliable clinical guidelines for most affected patients, the criteria listed may not be feasible for all patients [14,15]. In particular, diagnosis of both acute and chronic PJI is complicated in patients with rheumatoid arthritis where aseptic joint inflammation causes similar clinical and laboratory presentation. Qin et al. recently demonstrated that commonly used laboratory markers of non-operated rheumatoid arthritis patients do not differ significantly to those of patients with chronic PJI [19]. Patients with active rheumatoid arthritis of the operated joint are always scored to be likely affected by PJI. There is a paucity of data on differentiating PJI from rheumatoid arthritis in patients with previous knee or hip arthroplasty. While PJI cannot be ruled out with current diagnostic standards, a more detailed understanding of the relevant serum and synovial marker levels is necessary to personalize diagnostics and avoid unnecessary surgical intervention.

In this study, we retrospectively analyzed the cases of 17 patients with rheumatoid arthritis and 121 patients with no diagnosed rheumatoid disease who underwent surgical intervention due to microbiology-positive PJI of the hip or knee joint. This is the first study to evaluate differences in serum and synovial fluid markers in patients affected by this pathology.

2. Materials and Methods

2.1. Patients

This study was approved by the Charité University hospital ethics board (EA2/083/19) and was completed in accordance with the Declaration of Helsinki.

All patients receiving total knee or hip replacement exchange surgery due to acute or chronic PJI between 2013 and 2021 at the Charité university hospital in Berlin, Germany were retrospectively analyzed in this study. Patients were treated in a specialized department using a centralized and interdisciplinary treatment approach. In total, we analyzed patient files of 138 patients.

Inclusion criteria were a previously implanted knee or hip replacement and diagnosed PJI. As rheumatoid arthritis and PJI share clinical and paraclinical features, PJI was defined according to modified EBJIS criteria [20]: microbiological growth in synovial fluid, two or more tissue samples (for highly virulent organisms or in patients being treated with antibiotics, one positive sample confirmed infection), or sonication fluid (>50 CFU/mL) and at least one of the following criteria: (1) prevalence of a sinus tract or purulence around a component; (2) >2000 leukocytes/µL or >70% granulocytes in the synovial fluid; or (3) histology of intra-operatively acquired tissue Krenn and Morawietz type II or type III [21]. Acute PJI was defined as an infection within 4 weeks after primary arthroplasty surgery or acute onset of PJI-related symptoms less than 4 weeks before diagnosis and treatment of PJI. Symptom onset >4 weeks was classified as chronic PJI.

Rheumatoid arthritis was diagnosed prior to occurrence of PJI by a board-certified rheumatologist according to the ACR/EULAR Classification Criteria [22]. All patients were actively treated by a rheumatologist.

Patients who met one or more of the following criteria were excluded from this study: (1) culture-negative patients meeting EBJIS criteria for PJI; or (2) primary knee or hip joint infection without prosthesis. There were no further exclusions.

The enrolled patient population was divided into two groups based on whether patients diagnosed with rheumatoid disease (group A) or not (group B). Both groups were subdivided into acute and chronic cases: A1, acute cases with immune disorders; A2, chronic cases with immune disorders; B1, acute cases without immune disorders; B2, chronic cases without immune disorders.

Besides clinical and paraclinical examination, we assessed demographic data including age, BMI, ASA score, the number of prior surgeries on the affected knee or hip, pathological classification of tissue specimens, and laboratory results.

2.2. Statistical Analysis

All data were collected and recorded in Microsoft® Excel® 2016 (version 2111 Build 16.0.14701.20240, Microsoft, Redmond, WA USA). Continuous data were presented as median and IQR and analyzed using Student's t test or Mann–Whitney U test where applicable. Data between two groups were compared using chi-square test. Optimal cut-off values were determined using the Youden index (J) method (maximal value of "sensitivity + specificity-1") [23]. Based on cut-offs, sensitivity and specificity were defined and NPV, PPV, ROC, and AUC determined. Survival analysis was presented through Kaplan–Meier survival curves. All statistical analyses and plots were analyzed using R software (version: 3.6.3. R Development Core Team, Vienna, Austria).

3. Results

3.1. Patient Characteristics

Patient characteristics are outlined in Table 1. In total, 138 patients were enrolled in this study: 17 patients with rheumatoid arthritis and PJI (group A) and 121 patients without rheumatoid arthritis and PJI (group B). Of the patients included in our analysis, 76 were male (group A: 12; group B: 64) and 62 were female (group A: 5; group B: 57). Average patient age was 72.94 ± 7.10 years in group A and 69.07 ± 10.83. Mean BMI was 29.83 ± 6.97 for group A and 30.59 ± 5.82 for group B. Most patients had an ASA score of 2 (17.65% group A; 56.20% group B) or 3 (70.59% group A; 36.36% group B). Acute PJI occurred in 9 (52.94%; group A) and 54 (44.63%; group B) patients, and chronic PJI in 8 (47.06%; group A) and 67 (55.37%; group B) patients. Most patients had more than one revision surgery prior to PJI (70.59% in group A; 61.98% in group B). No significant differences for any of the analyzed parameters were found.

Table 1. Patient Characteristics.

	Group A (Rheumatoid Arthritis Patients)	Group B (without Rheumatoid Arthritis Patients)	p Value
Sex			
Male [# (%)]	12 (70.59%)	64 (52.89%)	0.17
Female [# (%)]	5 (29.41%)	57 (47.11%)	
BMI [kg/m^2]	29.83 ± 6.97	30.59 ± 5.82	0.69
Age [years]	72.94 ± 7.10	69.07 ± 10.83	0.06
PJI onset			
Acute [# (%)]	9 (52.94%)	54 (44.63%)	0.52
Chronic [# (%)]	8 (47.06%)	67 (55.37%)	
ASA score			
1 [# (%)]	0 (0.00%)	2 (1.65%)	0.06
2 [# (%)]	3 (17.65%)	68 (56.20%)	
3 [# (%)]	12 (70.59%)	44 (36.36%)	
4 [# (%)]	1 (5.88%)	4 (3.31%)	
5 [# (%)]	0 (0.00%)	1 (0.83%)	
Number of prior revision surgeries			
One [# (%)]	5 (29.41%)	46 (38.02%)	0.49
More than one [# (%)]	12 (70.59%)	75 (61.98%)	

#, number of patients.

3.2. Pathology and Microbiology

Pathology results indicated an infection (Krenn and Morawietz score of 2 or 3) in 88.24% of the patients with rheumatoid arthritis (group A) and in 77.69% of the patients without rheumatoid arthritis (group B; $p = 0.32$). Of these, 66.67% (group A) and 55.32% (group B) had a low-grade infection and 33.33% (group A) and 44.68% (group B) had a high-grade infection ($p = 0.41$). The remaining patients had a Krenn and Morawietz score of 1 or 4: 11.76% in group A and 22.31% in group B. In none of the patients analyzed was a sinus tract prevalent.

For all patients, synovial fluid samples were analyzed for pathogens (Table 2). In both groups, *Staphylococcus aureus* (47.06% in group A, 33.06% in group B) followed by *Staphylococcus epidermidis* (35.29% in group A, 19.83% in group B) had the highest incidence rate.

Table 2. Pre- and perioperative pathogens.

Pathogen	Group A (Rheumatoid Arthritis Patients)	Group B (without Rheumatoid Arthritis Patients)
Staphylococcus aureus	8 (47.06%)	40 (33.06%)
Staphylococcus epidermidis	6 (35.29%)	24 (19.83%)
Cutibacterium acnes	-	12 (9.91%)
Enteroccocus faecalis	1 (5.88%)	10 (8.26%)
Streptococcus anginosus	1 (5.88%)	2 (1.65%)
Streptococcus dysgalactiae	1 (5.88%)	8 (6.61%)
Escherichia coli	-	7 (5.79%)
Staphylococcus hominis	-	8 (6.61%)
Candida albicans	-	1 (0.83%)
Candida parapsilosis	-	2 (1.65%)
Cutibacterium avidum	-	1 (0.83%)
Staphylococcus capitis	-	2 (1.65%)
Streptococcus agalactiae	-	1 (0.83%)
Streptococcus mitis	-	1 (0.83%)
Streptococcus pyogenes	-	1 (0.83%)
Streptococcus pneumoniae	-	1 (0.83%)

3.3. Laboratory

Peripheral blood CRP concentration and WBC numbers as well as synovial fluid cell counts were analyzed for all patients. For acute PJI, no significant difference between patients with (group A1) and without rheumatoid arthritis (group B1) were found (Table 3): Median CRP was 88.00 and 129.45 mg/L ($p = 0.92$), WBC count 9.13 and 9.93 cells/nL ($p = 0.30$), synovial WBC 60.75 and 48.92 cells/nL ($p = 0.54$), and synovial PMN cell count 55.89 and 48.24 cells/nL ($p = 0.74$), respectively. All parameters analyzed showed high variability.

In patients with chronic PJI, peripheral blood CRP (group A2: 43.25 versus B2: 18.80 mg/L; $p = 0.05$), synovial WBC count (group A2: 34.68 versus B2: 8.33 cells/nL; $p = 0.02$), synovial monocyte cell count (group A2: 2.27 versus B2: 0.79 cells/nL; $p = 0.04$), and synovial PMN cell count (group A2: 33.36 versus B2: 6.13 cells/nL; $p = 0.02$) were significantly elevated in patients with rheumatoid arthritis (Table 3). In contrast, peripheral blood WBC count did not differ significantly (group A2: 6.86 versus B2: 7.45 cells/nL; $p = 0.75$).

ROC analysis was conducted for the analyzed parameters: AUC, best cut-off values, sensitivity, specificity, and NPV and PPV are listed in Table 4. All analyzed parameters showed poor discrimination for patients with acute PJI. Conversely, in patients with chronic PJI serum CRP levels (AUC = 0.71), synovial WBC count (AUC = 0.78), synovial monocyte cell count (AUC = 0.75), and synovial percentage of PMN cell count (AUC = 0.71) showed acceptable discrimination and synovial PMN cell count (AUC = 0.80) showed excellent discrimination (Figure 1). While for any of these parameters, sensitivity and NPV was above 75% and 95%, respectively, specificity and PPV only ranged from 55% to 74% and 18% to 26%, respectively.

Table 3. Laboratory results before prosthesis explantation.

	Group A1 (Rheumatoid Arthritis Patients; n = 9)		Group B1 (without Rheumatoid Arthritis Patients; n = 54)			
	Median	IQR	Median	IQR	W	p Value
Acute PJI						
Serum CRP [mg/L]	88.00	86.90–256.20	129.45	72.03–244.22	237	0.92
Peripheral blood WBC count [cells/nL]	9.13	6.17–12.03	9.93	7.22–14.22	190	0.30
Synovial WBC count [cells/nL]	60.75	54.72–118.06	48.92	33.58–197.56	178	0.54
Synovial monocyte cell count [cells/nL]	6.69	2.21–11.43	3.97	2.05–13.85	136	0.93
Synovial PMN cell count [cells/nL]	55.89	48.41–86.94	48.24	31.30–160.93	144	0.74
Synovial percentage of monocytes [%]	0.11	0.04–0.12	0.09	0.05–0.16	120	0.69
Synovial percentage of PMN cells [%]	0.89	0.88–0.96	0.91	0.84–0.95	149	0.62
	Group A2 (Rheumatoid Arthritis Patients; n = 8)		Group B2 (without Rheumatoid Arthritis Patients; n = 67)			
	Median	IQR	Median	IQR	W	p Value
Chronic PJI						
Serum CRP [mg/L]	43.25	25.02–145.00	18.80	6.45–47.15	372	0.05
Peripheral blood WBC count [cells/nL]	6.86	5.16–10.81	7.45	6.25–8.39	245	0.75
Synovial WBC count [cells/nL]	34.68	23.06–103.17	8.33	0.86–23.37	258	0.02
Synovial monocyte cell count [cells/nL]	2.27	1.16–13.5	0.79	0.33–2.28	244	0.04
Synovial PMN cell count [cells/nL]	33.36	20.48–70.75	6.13	0.43–16.68	260	0.02
Synovial percentage of monocytes [%]	0.10	0.05–0.15	0.23	0.08–0.43	102	0.13
Synovial percentage of PMN cells [%]	0.90	0.85–0.95	0.77	0.55–0.91	234	0.09

Table 4. Diagnostic value analysis.

	Cut-Off	Sensitivity	Specificity	NPV	PPV	AUC	AUC CI
Acute PJI							
Serum CRP [mg/L]	107.65	33.30%	38.90%	77.80%	8.30%	0.51	0.31–0.70
Peripheral Blood WBC count [cells/nL]	13.36	16.80%	63.00%	79.10%	8.40%	0.61	0.43–0.78
Synovial WBC count [cells/nL]	43.18	100%	35.90%	100%	24.20%	0.57	0.41–0.73
Synovial monocyte cell count [cells/nL]	2.06	100%	26.30%	100%	20.00%	0.51	0.30–0.71
Synovial PMN cell count [cells/nL]	37.79	100%	31.60%	100%	21.20%	0.54	0.37–0.70
Synovial percentage of monocytes [%]	10.07	57.10%	63.20%	88.90%	22.20%	0.45	0.20–0.69
Synovial percentage of PMN cells [%]	0.90	100%	9.30%	100%	15.60%	0.44	0.20–0.69

Table 4. Cont.

	Cut-Off	Sensitivity	Specificity	NPV	PPV	AUC	AUC CI
Chronic PJI							
Serum CRP [mg/L]	29.05	75.00%	60.60%	95.20%	18.80%	0.71	0.50–0.90
Peripheral Blood WBC count [cells/nL]	5.495	62.50%	10.60%	70.00%	7.80%	0.54	0.23–0.83
Synovial WBC count [cells/nL]	19.48	83.30%	72.70%	97.60%	25.00%	0.78	0.61–0.95
Synovial monocyte cell count [cells/nL]	0.83	100%	55.60%	100%	20.00%	0.75	0.58–0.92
Synovial PMN cell count [cells/nL]	16.18	83.30%	74.10%	97.60%	26.30%	0.80	0.63–0.96
Synovial percentage of monocytes [%]	14.70	16.70%	41.80%	82.10%	3.00%	0.69	0.50–0.87
Synovial percentage of PMN cells [%]	85.30	83.30%	73.00%	97.10%	18.50%	0.71	0.52–0.90

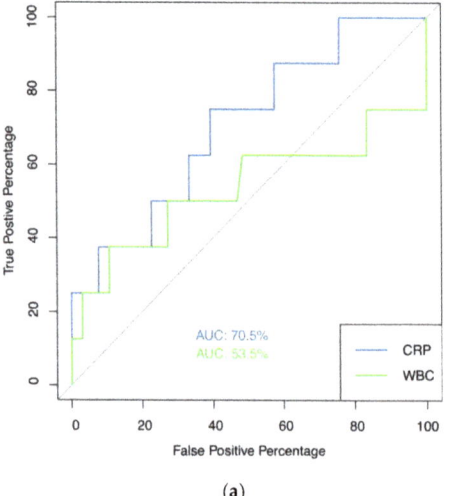
(a)

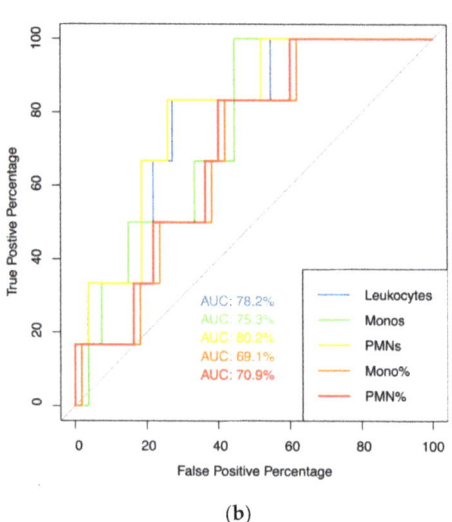
(b)

Figure 1. AUC Analysis. (**a**) AUC analysis for serum CRP (blue line) and peripheral blood WBC count (green line) in patients with chronic PJI; (**b**) AUC analysis for synovial fluid WBC count (blue line), monocyte cell count (green line), PMN cell count (yellow line), synovial percentage of monocytes (orange line), and percentage of PMN cell count (red line).

3.4. Prosthesis Survival

Risk for prosthesis failure due to recurrent PJI or aseptic loosening (Figure 2) was significantly elevated in patients with rheumatoid arthritis (prosthesis survival rate in group A: 78.07% versus group B: 52.94%; $p = 0.03$). Additionally, median prosthesis survival times were significantly shorter in group A (median: 1 year, IQR: 1.00–3.00 years) compared to group B (median: 2 years, IQR: 1.75–4.00 years; $p = 0.05$).

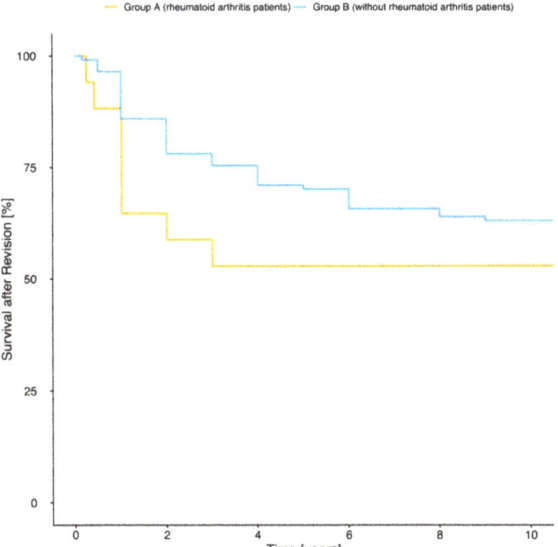

Figure 2. Prosthesis survival rate. Diagnosed recurrent PJI or aseptic loosening was classified as prosthesis failure. After 9 years, 47.06% of patients with rheumatoid arthritis (blue line) and 21.93% of patients without rheumatoid arthritis (yellow line) had suffered from prosthesis failure.

4. Discussion

In this study, we analyzed differences in clinical patient characteristics, laboratory parameters, and prosthesis survival rates in patients with and without rheumatoid arthritis and acute or chronic PJI. Additionally, we retrospectively evaluated the capability of laboratory markers to distinguish these patient groups. Long-term revision arthroplasty failure rate was significantly elevated in patients with rheumatoid arthritis and PJI compared to patients without autoimmune disease.

In both acute and chronic PJI, attending physicians are challenged to accurately confirm diagnosis in patients that are presenting with clinical features of PJI. Similar clinical and laboratory features of aseptic joint inflammation in patients with rheumatoid arthritis and arthroplasty significantly complicate the diagnosis of PJI. All patients with symptoms of active autoimmune arthritis after primary arthroplasty are classified as PJI-likely cases [14,15]. Inherently, investigations are limited to positive cases as PJI-negative cases in patients with active rheumatoid arthritis do not exist per definition. Commonly, diagnosis relies upon peripheral blood WBC count and serum CRP, as well as synovial WBC count and PMN cell percentage [13–15]. Establishing the diagnosis is challenging as guidelines were derived from PJI patients without rheumatoid arthritis [24]. Previous research reported the risk of infection in patients with rheumatoid arthritis to be significantly increased [7,25], potentially due to anti-rheumatic immunosuppressive therapy [26]. However, Trikha et al. found rheumatoid arthritis not to be an independent risk-factor for PJI in a murine model [27], suggesting PJI may be falsely diagnosed in some patients. Thus, in our study, only culture-positive patients were included to avoid analysis of false-positive cases.

To initiate treatment and avoid short- and long-term complications such as sepsis, recurrent PJI or aseptic loosening, a diagnosis is often needed in a short time frame. While microbiological culture is essential, it is not feasible in an acute setting due to culture time [16] and may be negative despite the presence of PJI [17,18]. In our study, we did not find good discriminatory power for peripheral blood WBC counts, serum CRP, synovial WBC count, synovial PNM cell count, synovial percentage of PNM cells, or synovial percentage of monocytes in acute PJI. While discriminatory power for these parameters was good to excellent in chronic PJI, specificity and PPV were only between 55% and 74% and 18% and 26%, respectively. Novel diagnostic serum and synovial markers such as alpha-defensin, soluble tumor necrosis factor receptor, and B-cell activating factor, as well as technologies such as next-generation sequencing, promise to improve current standards [18,28,29] and could especially benefit rheumatoid arthritis patients.

Due to the immediate severe impact on patients' life quality and to avoid unnecessary surgery, particular consideration must be given to false-positive diagnoses [30,31]. Rheumatoid arthritis patients are especially at risk as improvement of quality of life has been found to be poorer compared to patients with osteoarthritis after primary total joint replacement [32]. In our study, we found prosthesis failure rates after revision arthroplasty to be significantly elevated in patients with rheumatoid arthritis, further stressing the need for a more personalized diagnostic and therapeutic approach in these patients. Similarly, prosthesis survival rates after revision arthroplasty have been found to be significantly decreased in non-rheumatoid arthritis patients [11,12,33].

Limitations of the current study include the heterogeneity of the analyzed population, the retrospective study design, the analyzed rheumatoid arthritis cohort size, and the exclusion of potentially PJI-positive but culture-negative cases with potential subsequent statistical bias.

In conclusion, the current guidelines and routinely used laboratory markers have limited utility in distinguishing acute PJI in rheumatoid patients. In cases with suspected chronic PJI but low levels of serum CRP and synovial cell markers, physicians should consider the possibility of activated autoimmune arthritis. The observed elevated prosthesis failure rate in these patients stresses the need for novel diagnostic markers and a more personalized diagnostic and therapeutic approach for affected patients.

Author Contributions: Conceptualization, A.K., C.G. and C.P.; Data curation, Y.R. and L.B.; Formal analysis, Y.R. and A.K.; Investigation, Y.R., L.B. and A.K.; Methodology, Y.R. and A.K.; Supervision, C.G., C.P. and A.K.; Validation, L.B. and A.K.; Visualization, Y.R.; Writing—original draft, Y.R. and A.K.; Writing—review and editing, A.K. All authors have read and agreed to the published version of the manuscript.

Funding: The authors indicated that no external funding was received for any aspect of this work.

Institutional Review Board Statement: This study was approved by the local ethics board (EA2/083/19) and was performed in accordance with the Declaration of Helsinki.

Data Availability Statement: All data presented in this study are available on request from the corresponding author.

Acknowledgments: Arne Kienzle is participant in the BIH-Charité Junior Clinician Scientist Program funded by the Charité—Universitätsmedizin Berlin and the Berlin Institute of Health.

Conflicts of Interest: The authors declare no conflict of interest.

Abbreviations

American Society of Anesthesiologists, ASA; area under curve, AUC; body mass index, BMI; C-reaction protein, CRP; interquartile range, IQR; negative predictive values, NPV; periprosthetic joint infection, PJI; polymorphonuclear, PMN; positive predictive values, PPV; receiver operating curve, ROC; white blood cell, WBC.

References

1. Delanois, R.E.; Mistry, J.B.; Gwam, C.U.; Mohamed, N.S.; Choksi, U.S.; Mont, M.A. Current Epidemiology of Revision Total Knee Arthroplasty in the United States. *J. Arthroplast.* **2017**, *32*, 2663–2668. [CrossRef] [PubMed]
2. Kurtz, S.M.; Lau, E.; Schmier, J.; Ong, K.L.; Zhao, K.; Parvizi, J. Infection Burden for Hip and Knee Arthroplasty in the United States. *J. Arthroplast.* **2008**, *23*, 984–991. [CrossRef] [PubMed]
3. Kapadia, B.H.; Berg, R.A.; Daley, J.A.; Fritz, J.; Bhave, A.; Mont, M.A. Periprosthetic joint infection. *Lancet* **2016**, *387*, 386–394. [CrossRef]

4. Zimmerli, W.; Trampuz, A.; Ochsner, P.E. Prosthetic-joint infections. *N. Engl. J. Med.* **2004**, *351*, 1645–1654. [CrossRef]
5. Huotari, K.; Peltola, M.; Jamsen, E. The incidence of late prosthetic joint infections: A registry-based study of 112,708 primary hip and knee replacements. *Acta Orthop.* **2015**, *86*, 321–325. [CrossRef]
6. Insall, J.N.; Thompson, F.M.; Brause, B.D. Two-stage reimplantation for the salvage of infected total knee arthroplasty. *J. Bone Jt. Surg.* **1983**, *65*, 1087–1098. [CrossRef]
7. Poss, R.; Thornhill, T.S.; Ewald, F.C.; Thomas, W.H.; Batte, N.J.; Sledge, C.B. Factors influencing the incidence and outcome of infection following total joint arthroplasty. *Clin. Orthop. Relat. Res.* **1984**, *182*, 117–126. [CrossRef]
8. Argenson, J.N.; Arndt, M.; Babis, G.; Battenberg, A.; Budhiparama, N.; Catani, F.; Chen, F.; de Beaubien, B.; Ebied, A.; Esposito, S.; et al. Hip and Knee Section, Treatment, Debridement and Retention of Implant: Proceedings of International Consensus on Orthopedic Infections. *J. Arthroplast.* **2019**, *34*, S399–S419. [CrossRef]
9. Nace, J.; Siddiqi, A.; Talmo, C.T.; Chen, A.F. Diagnosis and Management of Fungal Periprosthetic Joint Infections. *J. Am. Acad. Orthop. Surg.* **2019**, *27*, e804–e818. [CrossRef]
10. Kuiper, J.W.; Rustenburg, C.M.; Willems, J.H.; Verberne, S.J.; Peters, E.J.; Saouti, R. Results and Patient Reported Outcome Measures (PROMs) after One-Stage Revision for Periprosthetic Joint Infection of the Hip: A Single-centre Retrospective Study. *J. Bone Jt. Infect.* **2018**, *3*, 143–149. [CrossRef]
11. Kienzle, A.; Walter, S.; Palmowski, Y.; Kirschbaum, S.; Biedermann, L.; von Roth, P.; Perka, C.; Müller, M. Influence of Gender on Occurrence of Aseptic Loosening and Recurrent PJI after Revision Total Knee Arthroplasty. *Osteology* **2021**, *1*, 92–104. [CrossRef]
12. Kienzle, A.; Walter, S.; Von Roth, P.; Fuchs, M.; Winkler, T.; Müller, M. High Rates of Aseptic Loosening After Revision Total Knee Arthroplasty for Periprosthetic Joint Infection. *JBJS Open Access* **2020**, *5*, e20.00026. [CrossRef] [PubMed]
13. Goswami, K.; Parvizi, J.; Maxwell Courtney, P. Current Recommendations for the Diagnosis of Acute and Chronic PJI for Hip and Knee-Cell Counts, Alpha-Defensin, Leukocyte Esterase, Next-generation Sequencing. *Curr. Rev. Musculoskelet. Med.* **2018**, *11*, 428–438. [CrossRef] [PubMed]
14. Parvizi, J.; Tan, T.L.; Goswami, K.; Higuera, C.; Della Valle, C.; Chen, A.F.; Shohat, N. The 2018 Definition of Periprosthetic Hip and Knee Infection: An Evidence-Based and Validated Criteria. *J. Arthroplast.* **2018**, *33*, 1309–1314.e2. [CrossRef] [PubMed]
15. McNally, M.; Sousa, R.; Wouthuyzen-Bakker, M.; Chen, A.F.; Soriano, A.; Vogely, H.C.; Clauss, M.; Higuera, C.A.; Trebše, R. The EBJIS definition of periprosthetic joint infection. *Bone Jt. J.* **2021**, *103-B*, 18–25. [CrossRef] [PubMed]
16. Talsma, D.; Ploegmakers, J.; Jutte, P.; Kampinga, G.; Wouthuyzen-Bakker, M. Time to positivity of acute and chronic periprosthetic joint infection cultures. *Diagn. Microbiol. Infect. Dis.* **2021**, *99*, 115178. [CrossRef]
17. Palan, J.; Nolan, C.; Sarantos, K.; Westerman, R.; King, R.; Foguet, P. Culture-negative periprosthetic joint infections. *EFORT Open Rev.* **2019**, *4*, 585–594. [CrossRef]
18. Tarabichi, M.; Shohat, N.; Goswami, K.; Alvand, A.; Silibovsky, R.; Belden, K.; Parvizi, J. Diagnosis of Periprosthetic Joint Infection: The Potential of Next-Generation Sequencing. *J. Bone Jt. Surg.* **2018**, *100*, 147–154. [CrossRef]
19. Qin, L.; Wang, H.; Zhao, C.; Chen, C.; Chen, H.; Li, X.; Wang, J.; Hu, N.; Huang, W. Serum and Synovial Biomarkers for Distinguishing Between Chronic Periprosthetic Joint Infections and Rheumatoid Arthritis: A Prospective Cohort Study. *J. Arthroplast.* **2021**, *37*, 342–346. [CrossRef]
20. Ochsner, P.E.; Borens, O.; Bodler, P.-M. *Infections of the Musculoskeletal System: Basic Principles, Prevention, Diagnosis and Treatment*; Swiss Orthopaedics In-House-Publisher: Grandvaux, Switzerland, 2014.
21. Krenn, V.; Morawietz, L.; Perino, G.; Kienapfel, H.; Ascherl, R.; Hassenpflug, G.; Thomsen, M.; Thomas, P.; Huber, M.; Kendoff, D.; et al. Revised histopathological consensus classification of joint implant related pathology. *Pathol. Res. Pract.* **2014**, *210*, 779–786. [CrossRef]
22. Kay, J.; Upchurch, K.S. ACR/EULAR 2010 rheumatoid arthritis classification criteria. *Rheumatology* **2012**, *51* (Suppl. 6), vi5–vi9. [CrossRef] [PubMed]
23. Youden, W.J. Index for rating diagnostic tests. *Cancer* **1950**, *3*, 32–35. [CrossRef]
24. Premkumar, A.; Morse, K.; Levack, A.E.; Bostrom, M.P.; Carli, A.V. Periprosthetic Joint Infection in Patients with Inflammatory Joint Disease: Prevention and Diagnosis. *Curr. Rheumatol. Rep.* **2018**, *20*, 68. [CrossRef] [PubMed]
25. Stundner, O.; Danninger, T.; Chiu, Y.-L.; Sun, X.; Goodman, S.M.; Russell, L.A.; Figgie, M.; Mazumdar, M.; Memtsoudis, S.G. Rheumatoid Arthritis vs Osteoarthritis in Patients Receiving Total Knee Arthroplasty: Perioperative Outcomes. *J. Arthroplast.* **2014**, *29*, 308–313. [CrossRef] [PubMed]
26. Yeganeh, M.H.; Kheir, M.M.; Shahi, A.; Parvizi, J. Rheumatoid Arthritis, Disease Modifying Agents, and Periprosthetic Joint Infection: What Does a Joint Surgeon Need to Know? *J. Arthroplasty.* **2018**, *33*, 1258–1264. [CrossRef] [PubMed]
27. Trikha, R.; Greig, D.; Sekimura, T.; Cevallos, N.; Kelley, B.; Mamouei, Z.; Hart, C.; Ralston, M.; Turkmani, A.; Sassoon, A.; et al. Active rheumatoid arthritis in a mouse model is not an independent risk factor for periprosthetic joint infection. *PLoS ONE* **2021**, *16*, e0250910. [CrossRef]
28. Indelli, P.F.; Ghirardelli, S.; Violante, B.; Amanatullah, D.F. Next generation sequencing for pathogen detection in periprosthetic joint infections. *EFORT Open Rev.* **2021**, *6*, 236–244. [CrossRef]
29. Keemu, H.; Vaura, F.; Maksimow, A.; Maksimow, M.; Jokela, A.; Hollmén, M.; Mäkelä, K. Novel Biomarkers for Diagnosing Periprosthetic Joint Infection from Synovial Fluid and Serum. *JBJS Open Access* **2021**, *6*, e20.00067. [CrossRef]
30. Patil, S.; Garbuz, D.S.; Greidanus, N.V.; Masri, B.; Duncan, C.P. Quality of Life Outcomes in Revision vs Primary Total Hip Arthroplasty: A Prospective Cohort Study. *J. Arthroplast.* **2008**, *23*, 550–553. [CrossRef]

31. Greidanus, N.V.; Peterson, R.C.; Masri, B.; Garbuz, D.S. Quality of Life Outcomes in Revision Versus Primary Total Knee Arthroplasty. *J. Arthroplast.* **2011**, *26*, 615–620. [CrossRef]
32. Dusad, A.; Pedro, S.; Mikuls, T.R.; Hartman, C.W.; Garvin, K.L.; O'Dell, J.R.; Michaud, K. Impact of Total Knee Arthroplasty as Assessed Using Patient-Reported Pain and Health-Related Quality of Life Indices: Rheumatoid Arthritis Versus Osteoarthritis. *Arthritis Rheumatol.* **2015**, *67*, 2503–2511. [CrossRef] [PubMed]
33. Karczewski, D.; Ren, Y.; Andronic, O.; Akgün, D.; Perka, C.; Müller, M.; Kienzle, A. Candida periprosthetic joint infections—Risk factors and outcome between albicans and non-albicans strains. *Int. Orthop.* **2022**, *46*, 449–456. [CrossRef] [PubMed]

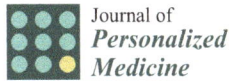

Journal of Personalized Medicine

Article

Automatic Segmentation for Favourable Delineation of Ten Wrist Bones on Wrist Radiographs Using Convolutional Neural Network

Bo-kyeong Kang [1,2,†], Yelin Han [3,†], Jaehoon Oh [2,4,*,‡], Jongwoo Lim [2,3,*,‡], Jongbin Ryu [5,6], Myeong Seong Yoon [2,4], Juncheol Lee [2,4] and Soorack Ryu [7]

1. Department of Radiology, College of Medicine, Hanyang University, Seoul 04763, Korea; msbbogri@hanyang.ac.kr
2. Machine Learning Research Center for Medical Data, Hanyang University, Seoul 04764, Korea; yoon5690@naver.com (M.S.Y.); doldoly@hanyang.ac.kr (J.L.)
3. Department of Computer Science, Hanyang University, 222 Wangsimni-ro, Seongdong-gu, Seoul 04763, Korea; gdf1845@gmail.com
4. Department of Emergency Medicine, College of Medicine, Hanyang University, 222 Wangsimni-ro, Seongdong-gu, Seoul 04763, Korea
5. Department of Software and Computer Engineering, Ajou University, Suwon 16499, Korea; jongbin.ryu@gmail.com
6. Department of Artificial Intelligence, Ajou University, Suwon 16499, Korea
7. Biostatistical Consulting and Research Lab, Medical Research Collaborating Center, Hanyang University, Seoul 04763, Korea; rsa4648@hanyang.ac.kr
* Correspondence: ojjai@hanyang.ac.kr (J.O.); jlim@hanyang.ac.kr (J.L.); Tel.: +82-2-2290-9829 (J.O.); Fax: +82-2-2290-9280 (J.O.)
† These authors contributed equally to this work.
‡ These authors contributed equally to this work.

Citation: Kang, B.-k.; Han, Y.; Oh, J.; Lim, J.; Ryu, J.; Yoon, M.S.; Lee, J.; Ryu, S. Automatic Segmentation for Favourable Delineation of Ten Wrist Bones on Wrist Radiographs Using Convolutional Neural Network. *J. Pers. Med.* **2022**, *12*, 776. https://doi.org/10.3390/jpm12050776

Academic Editors: Arne Kienzle and Henrik Bäcker

Received: 12 April 2022
Accepted: 10 May 2022
Published: 11 May 2022

Publisher's Note: MDPI stays neutral with regard to jurisdictional claims in published maps and institutional affiliations.

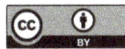

Copyright: © 2022 by the authors. Licensee MDPI, Basel, Switzerland. This article is an open access article distributed under the terms and conditions of the Creative Commons Attribution (CC BY) license (https://creativecommons.org/licenses/by/4.0/).

Abstract: Purpose: This study aimed to develop and validate an automatic segmentation algorithm for the boundary delineation of ten wrist bones, consisting of eight carpal and two distal forearm bones, using a convolutional neural network (CNN). Methods: We performed a retrospective study using adult wrist radiographs. We labeled the ground truth masking of wrist bones, and propose that the Fine Mask R-CNN consisted of wrist regions of interest (ROI) using a Single-Shot Multibox Detector (SSD) and segmentation via Mask R-CNN, plus the extended mask head. The primary outcome was an improvement in the prediction of delineation via the network combined with ground truth masking, and this was compared between two networks through five-fold validations. Results: In total, 702 images were labeled for the segmentation of ten wrist bones. The overall performance (mean (SD) of Dice coefficient) of the auto-segmentation of the ten wrist bones improved from 0.93 (0.01) using Mask R-CNN to 0.95 (0.01) using Fine Mask R-CNN ($p < 0.001$). The values of each wrist bone were higher when using the Fine Mask R-CNN than when using the alternative (all $p < 0.001$). The value derived for the distal radius was the highest, and that for the trapezoid was the lowest in both networks. Conclusion: Our proposed Fine Mask R-CNN model achieved good performance in the automatic segmentation of ten overlapping wrist bones derived from adult wrist radiographs.

Keywords: wrist; carpal bone; segmentation; deep learning; CNN

1. Introduction

Acute wrist pain related to trauma or non-trauma causes is a common complaint presented in primary care and emergency rooms [1,2]. Imaging is often necessary to make a definitive diagnosis of wrist pain, along with access to a clear history and physical examination, because no predetermined decision is possible. Standard plain radiographs are used as the initial diagnostic radiologic evaluation for most patients with wrist pain [3–5]. However, it is difficult for physicians—even an experienced radiologist—to accurately identify each bone contour, and to interpret subtle changes, because the wrist is composed of ten bones—eight carpal bones (trapezium, trapezoid, capitate, hamate, pisiform, triquetrum, lunate, and scaphoid) and two long bones (distal radius and distal ulna)—that overlap each other [4,5] (Figure 1a). Although wrist radiographs provide limited information, due to the limitations of projection views and clinical observations, they still offer crucial support for diagnostic and therapeutic determination in clinical practice [3–6].

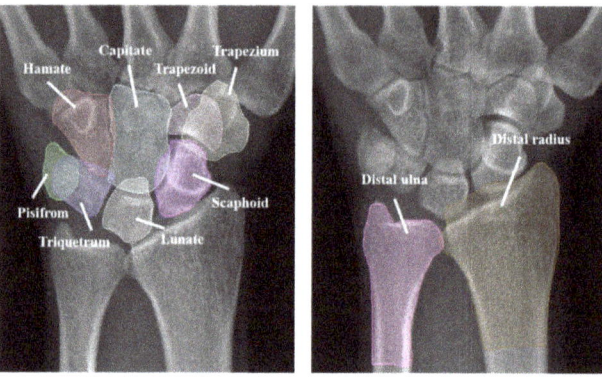

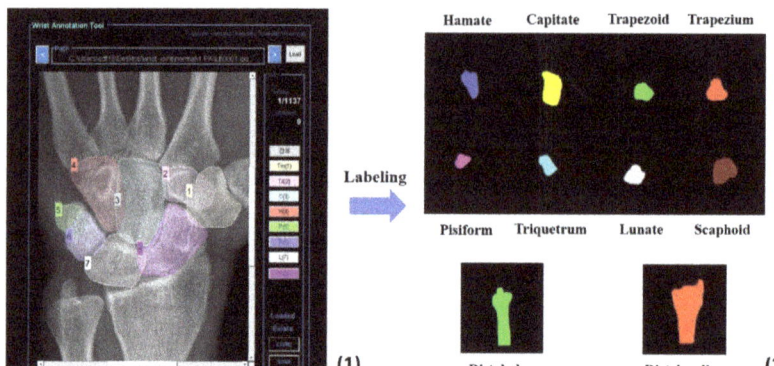

Figure 1. Anatomy and labeling of ten wrist bones on a wrist radiograph. (**a**) The anatomy of ten wrist bones, consisting of eight carpal bones and two distal forearm bones, on an anteroposterior radiograph. (**b**) Labeling process for the ground truth masking of wrist bones using a self-made customized tool. (**1**) The classification as one of ten wrist bones and the delineation of each bone's boundary; (**2**) Labeling and extraction of each bone.

Recently, the segmentation of bones using computer-aided algorithms has been studied for use in clinical diagnosis and treatment planning [7–10]. Wrist bone segmentation also has been studied as a predecessor to wrist fracture classification [11], bone age assessment [12,13], and the diagnosis of rheumatoid arthritis [14–16]. However, most wrist bone segmentation methods use conventional mathematical methods. Gou et al. conducted automatic segmentation through a dynamic programming algorithm [17], and Manos et al. employed the region growing [18] and region merging algorithms sequentially after pre-processing, using a Canny edge detector [19]. In addition, some advanced algorithms have been applied to overcome the disadvantages related to each medical image domain by combining these conventional methods [20,21].

Few studies of wrist bone segmentation via wrist radiograph, using deep learning, have been reported for reasons such as the low contrast between bone and tissue, the distances between the carpal bones, and the bones' irregular shapes. Moreover, there were fewer than ten wrist bones being segmented in these studies, because they were focused on bone age assessment in young children, whose wrist bones have not yet matured [22,23].

This study aimed to develop and validate an automatic segmentation algorithm for the prediction of the boundaries of ten wrist bones overlapping each other on an adult wrist radiograph, using a convolutional neural network.

2. Methods

2.1. Study Design

This was a retrospective study using wrist posteroanterior (PA) or anteroposterior (AP) radiographs, which were performed at one tertiary hospital (Seoul, Korea) between April 2020 and September 2021. This study was approved by the Institutional Review Board of Hanyang University Hospital, and the requirement for informed consent was waived by the IRBs of our hospital. All methods and procedures were carried out in accordance with the Declaration of Helsinki.

2.2. Dataset of Participants

We sorted and gathered wrist PA or AP radiographs from adult patients with wrist pain who visited the emergency room at the Hanyang University Hospital between January 2011 and December 2019. Their radiology reports stated "unremarkable study", "non-specific finding", or "no definite acute lesion". Radiographs were excluded when accurate delineation was impossible as a result of screws or other implants, the severe deformation of anatomical structures caused by acute fractures in another area, or past damage, malformation, or casts. Labeling for the ground truth masking of wrist bones was conducted with a program that was self-made and customized using a tool implemented in Matlab R2018b (MatLab, MathWorks, Natick, MA, USA), as shown in Figure 1b. The process was as follows: (1) classification as one of ten wrist bones; (2) delineation of each bone's boundary by two emergency physicians for segmentation; and (3) review and revision by a radiologist. Radiograph images were extracted using the picture archiving and communication system (PACS, PiView, INFINITT Healthcare, Seoul, Korea) as digital imaging and communication and medicine (DICOM)-format images, and stored in the Joint Photographic Experts Group (JPEG) format. No personal information was included in the images used for data collection, with personally identifying data excluded. In addition, arbitrary numbers were assigned to the images, which were then coded and managed.

2.3. Data Pre-Processing

We pre-processed our dataset via three methods in order to train our network stably. First, the wrist directions in all the training images were corrected to leftwards, as all right-hand wrist images were horizontally mirrored. This strategy eliminated wrist direction variations and unnecessary computations. Secondly, the sizes of the wrist radiography images were fixed, since the image size was different for every person. Finally, the input images were normalized, which is essential in order to effectively fine-tune the pre-trained Mask R-CNN (an object detection and segmentation simultaneously based on deep CNN) [24].

2.4. Network Architecture

The overall workflow of our method (Fine Mask R-CNN) for the automatic segmentation of wrist bones is illustrated in Figure 2a. It consists of two main steps—wrist region of interest (ROI) detection and segmentation.

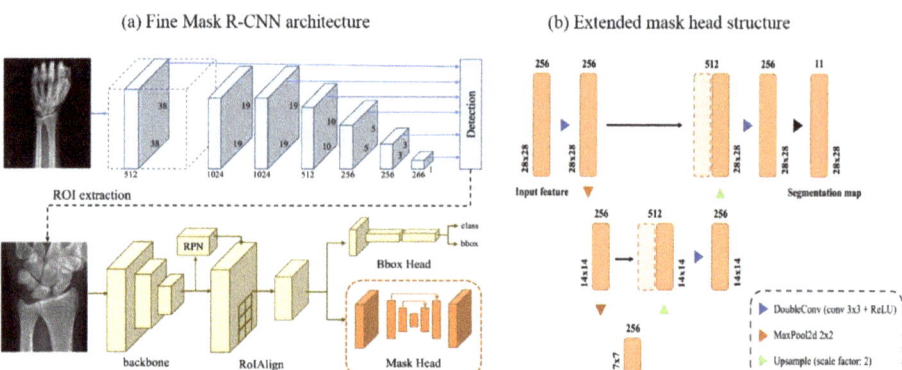

Figure 2. The Fine Mask R-CNN architecture. Our proposed network operates on a 2-stage method. (**a**) Detection of the regions of interest in the input wrist radiographs using SSD (blue) in the first stage and the delineation of 10 wrist bones using Mask R-CNN with the extended mask head in the second stage (yellow). (**b**) The structure of the extended mask head. This is an encoder–decoder structure, which can use previous information for the prediction of a specific part. ROI, region of interest; CNN, convolutional neural networks; SSD, Single-Shot Multibox Detector.

2.4.1. Wrist ROI Detection Model Using Single-Shot Multibox Detector (SSD)

In this paper, a specific region whose X-ray image only includes our target wrist bones is called the wrist ROI. The first stage is to detect the wrist ROI, then the segmentation model uses this detected wrist ROI as the input image. This cascade system can focus on this ROI and segment ten wrist bones more precisely, which could be helpful for our study, wherein the ROI is a small section of the overall image [25,26].

Here, we trained the Single-Shot Multibox Detector (SSD) [27], which is a network that performs object detection on all the feature maps of different sizes through multiple convolutional layers. Using these variously sized feature maps, SSD can detect small to large objects effectively. Training this detection network requires the ground truth bounding box of ROI, which we manually labeled according to the rule [23]. The size of the ROI is the average of 620 × 470 pixels, which is about one-third the size of the original image. This extracted ROI was re-scaled to 1820 × 1450 pixels, and then used as an input for the wrist segmentation model.

2.4.2. Wrist Segmentation Model Using Mask R-CNN with the Extended Mask Head

Most segmentation studies based on deep learning [7,28–30] have used the U-Net [31] architecture, which is the most popular algorithm for biomedical image segmentation. However, our proposed segmentation model was based on the Mask R-CNN [24], which is widely used for instance segmentation because most adult wrist bones overlap each other, especially the eight carpal bones. Therefore, some of the pixels could include two or more types of wrist bones.

In this paper, a finer segmentation network was proposed, which modified the mask head of the Mask R-CNN in two ways. Our first contribution to network design was a larger input size of the mask head. We used the 28 × 28 input feature, which is larger than the original, in the Mask R-CNN, as shown in Figure 2b. This advancement was motivated by the blurry contour problem mentioned in [32], which pointed out that the blurry contour appears as a result of a low-resolution regular grid of segmentation method. In other words, in the process of resizing the size of this coarse output to the original ROI size, the details nearby object boundaries were over-smoothing. We expect that a larger input size achieves better performance, but this will depend on the limitation of the hardware resource. Since we used the 28 × 28 input feature, the output probability map used for the segmentation model is 28 × 28 × 11, wherein 11 is the number of classes (ten wrist bones and background). We can prevent over-smoothing when interpolating the output probability map to the original image size by using this larger possibility map. This approach could be effective for use on the distal radius and distal ulna, because the resolution of these bones is greater than eight carpal bones. Additionally, we changed a mask head architecture from the original to an encoder–decoder structure, motivated by the U-Net, shown in Figure 2b. The structure of the U-Net connects multiple feature maps of different scales in an encoder–decoder architecture. With this architecture, high-resolution features can be combined with the upsampled features and more precise segmentation performance can be achieved than our baseline network, Mask R-CNN.

The weights of our proposed mask branch are updated similarly to those of the Mask R-CNN. A mask probability map $\hat{y}$ is computed using a per-pixel sigmoid function at each output pixel value. Then, the binary cross-entropy loss of each mask probability map $\hat{y}$ for N ROIs is computed. The final mask loss $L_{mask}(\hat{y})$ is computed as

$$BCE(y, \hat{y}) = -\sum_{i=1}^{2} [y_i log \hat{y}_i + (1 - y_i) log log (1 - \hat{y}_i)], \quad (1)$$

$$L_{mask}(\hat{y}) = \frac{1}{N} \sum_{k=1}^{N} BCE(y_{ck}, \hat{y_{ck}}), \quad (2)$$

where y_i is the ground truth class of either the bone or the background, and y_{ck} and $\hat{y_{ck}}$ are the ground truth and probability map corresponding to the predicted class of the kth ROI, respectively. Since the bone boundary is a very difficult region to correctly segment, the improvement of segmentation quality in the boundary region is a significant achievement, and offers much better results than visual observation.

2.4.3. Training and Validation of Automatic Segmentation Using Fine Mask R-CNN and Mask R-CNN

To ensure the consistency of our model, a five-fold cross-validation was employed in our experiments. With randomly divided wrist X-ray images into five parts, we used four out of five of which are used for training and the other for testing. Depending on which part we choose as the test dataset, we can have five different train/test dataset combinations. Therefore, we can train the five models with five different train and test datasets and analyze their outputs to ensure our model's robustness. In addition, this evaluation process can perform subject-based cross-validation by using all bones of one person used only for training or testing in one training phase.

Two networks were trained using a stochastic gradient descent (SGD) optimizer with a momentum equal to 0.9, and the initial learning rates were 0.001 and 0.0075, with weight decay factors of 0.0005 and 0.0001, respectively. The overall system employed the Pytorch library, and all the training and testing phases were performed on a GeForce GTX 1080 Ti GPU (NVIDIA, Santa Clara, CA, USA).

The baseline network and our proposed network were pre-trained by the ImageNet dataset and were fine-tuned with our collected wrist X-ray dataset. The fine-tuning algorithm transfers network parameters learned from a large common dataset to a specific task. Various studies have used a fine-tuning algorithm to analyze medical images, and its effectiveness has also been proven in the detection of other wrist fractures [33,34].

2.5. Primary Outcomes and Quantitative Evaluation

Our primary outcome was an improvement in the delineation predicted by networks in compliance with each wrist bone's ground truth masking. For the quantitative evaluation of performance, we used the Dice coefficient (Dice), a well-known area-based metric for evaluating segmentation algorithms. It estimates the degree of overlap between the ground truth area and the predicted area. The Dice coefficient is calculated as follows:

$$\text{Dice} = \frac{2\text{TP}}{2\text{TP} + \text{FP} + \text{FN}} \tag{3}$$

TP, FP and FN are the numbers of true positive, false positive, and false negative pixels, respectively. We measured the Dice coefficient for each bone, and calculated the average of 8 carpal bones, as well as the average Dice of 2 forearm bones and the total Dice of 10 bones to assess the overall performance of the model. This metric holds a value between 0 and 1, and higher values mean better predictions.

Additionally, we performed Turing tests on the ground truth masking performed by clinicians and the masking predicted by our network for the segmentation of ten wrist bones. The Turing test examines a machine's ability to exhibit intelligent behavior indistinguishable from, or equivalent to, that of a human. One professor and two residents at the department of radiology, who were not authors, were blinded as to the subject vis a vis masking; they scored between 1 (worst) and 5 (best) in terms of the quality of the delineation of the segmentation boundaries on the ground truth mask and the predicted mask of 140 images.

2.6. Visualization of Predicted Masking of Wrist Bones through Automatic Segmentation by Networks

The Dice coefficient used for quantitative evaluation in this paper is frequently used for segmentation model evaluations; however, it is an area-based metric, so it has a disadvantage in that it cannot evaluate the accuracy of boundaries. Therefore, we visualized the wrist bone segmentation results using networks in order to yield explainable and insightful analyses.

2.7. Statistical Analysis

The data were compiled using a standard spreadsheet application (Excel 2016; Microsoft, Redmond, WA, USA) and analyzed using NCSS 12 (Statistical Software 2018, NCSS, LLC. Kaysville, UT, USA, ncss.com/software/ncss). Kolmogorov–Smirnov tests were performed to demonstrate the normal distribution of all the datasets. We generated descriptive statistics, and here present them as frequency and percentage values in the categorical data, and as either median and interquartile range (IQR) (non-normal distribution) or mean and standard deviation (SD) (normal distribution). Paired *t*-tests or Wilcoxon signed rank tests were used to compare the performance between the Mask R-CNN as the baseline network and the Fine Mask R-CNN as the proposed network, and the Turing test was used to compare between the ground truth and the predicted mask. p-values < 0.05 were considered statistically significant. The intraclass correlation coefficient (ICC) was used to determine the agreement between three evaluators used in the Turing test. Values of ICC less than 0.5, between 0.5 and 0.75, between 0.75 and 0.9, and greater than 0.90 were indicative of poor, moderate, good, and excellent reliability, respectively [35].

3. Results

In total, 702 images were collected from 702 patients and all images were labeled for the annotation and segmentation of ten wrist bones. The baseline characteristics of participants who provided labeled images were 45.74 (16.66) years old, 53.30% female, and 69.42% images of the left wrist. 702 labeled images split 140 of set A, 140 of set B, 140 of Set C, 141 of set D, and 141 of set E. All images used for training both wrist ROI detection and segmentation model were through five-fold validation, and we obtained the test results of 702 images for our proposed models.

3.1. The Performance Test between the Fine Mask R-CNN and the Mask R-CNN for the Automatic Segmentation of Wrist Bones

The overall performance (mean [SD] of Dice) in the auto-segmentation of 10 wrist bones after training increased from 0.93 (0.01) via the Mask R-CNN to 0.95 (0.01) via the Fine Mask R-CNN ($p < 0.001$). All values for each bone were higher in the Fine Mask R-CNN than in the Mask R-CNN (all $p < 0.001$). The Dice value of the distal radius was the highest (0.96 (0.01)), and that of the trapezoid bone was the lowest (0.91 (0.05)) after training with the Fine Mask R-CNN, whereas the Dice value of the distal radius was the highest (0.94 (0.02)), and that of the trapezoid bone was the lowest value (0.90 (0.05)) after training with Mask R-CNN (Table 1).

3.2. The Turing Test between Ground Truth Masking by Clinicians and Masking Predicted by Fine Mask R-CNN for the Automatic Segmentation of Wrist Bones

The total scores (median [IQR]) of all ten wrist bones were 47 (38–50) via predicted masking and 48 (38–50) via predicted masking and 48 (41–50) via ground truth masking ($p < 0.001$). The evaluators estimated that the delineation of ground truth masking was better than that of predicted masking in each carpal bone (all $p < 0.001$), except for the trapezoid and scaphoid ($p = 0.25$, and $p = 0.39$ respectively). The scores of the distal radius and ulnar bones were also significantly different between the two masking methods (all $p < 0.001$). The ICC values amongst the evaluators were poor to moderate, in terms of both the ground truth and the predicted masking (Table 2).

3.3. Visualization of Predicted Masking for Wrist Bone Segmentation by Two Networks

The visualizations used for the delineation of eight carpal bones and two distal forearm segments, created by two different networks, are shown in Figure 3. Our proposed Fine Mask R-CNN achieves closer and more accurate delineation with ground truth masking than the other approach.

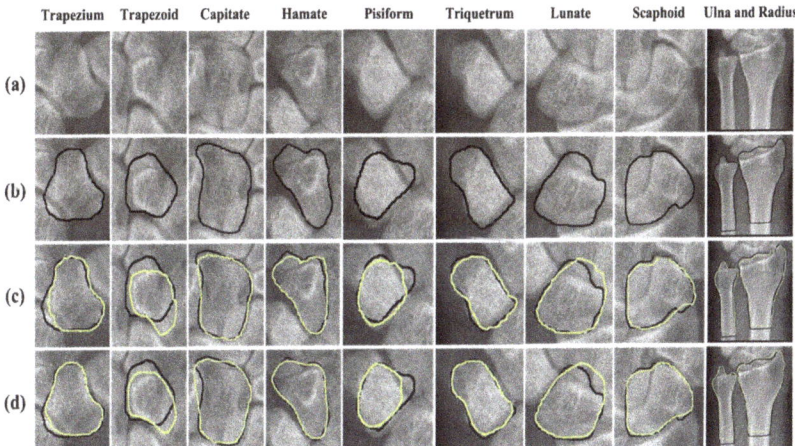

Figure 3. Visualization of Fine Mask R-CNN and Mask R-CNN network for the segmentation of ten wrist bones. (**a**) Original image of each wrist bone on the radiograph, (**b**) Delineation of segmented bone by physicians manually, (**c**) Delineation of segmented bone by Mask R-CNN, (**d**) Delineation of segmented bone by Fine Mask R-CNN with an extended mask head. Black lines indicate the ground truth masking segmented by physicians and yellow lines indicate the predicted masking segmented by CNN. CNN; convolutional neural networks.

Table 1. Comparison of the performance outcomes between the Mask R-CNN and the Fine Mask R-CNN for the automatic segmentation of ten wrist bones.

	Tm	Td	C	H	P	Tr	L	S	Carpal	R	U	Forearm	Total
Mask R-CNN Dice, mean [SD]	0.92 (0.03)	0.90 (0.05)	0.93 (0.04)	0.93 (0.02)	0.91 (0.05)	0.93 (0.02)	0.93 (0.02)	0.93 (0.02)	0.92 (0.01)	0.94 (0.02)	0.93 (0.02)	0.94 (0.01)	0.93 (0.01)
Fine Mask R-CNN Dice, mean [SD]	0.93 (0.03)	0.91 (0.05)	0.95 (0.04)	0.95 (0.02)	0.93 (0.04)	0.95 (0.02)	0.95 (0.02)	0.96 (0.02)	0.94 (0.01)	0.96 (0.01)	0.96 (0.02)	0.96 (0.01)	0.95 (0.01)
Comparison between two networks' *p*-values	<0.001 *	<0.001 *	<0.001 *	<0.001 *	<0.001 *	<0.001 *	<0.001 *	<0.001 *	<0.001 *	<0.001 *	<0.001 *	<0.001 *	<0.001 *

Dice, Dice coefficient; SD, standard deviation; Tm, trapezium; Td, trapezoid; C, capitate; H, hamate; P, pisiform; Tr, triquetrum; L, lunate; S, scaphoid; R, distal radius; U, distal ulna. Paired *t*-tests were used to compare the performance between two networks according to normality. * *p*-values < 0.05 were considered statistically significant.

Table 2. Result of the Turing test between the ground truth masking segmented by clinicians and the predicted masking segmented by Fine Mask R-CNN for the automatic segmentation of ten wrist bones.

			Tm	Td	C	H	P	Tr	L	S	Carpal	R	U	Forearm	Total
Prediction	Score	Median	4	5	4	5	5	5	5	5	37	5	5	10	47
		IQR	4, 5	5, 5	4, 5	4, 5	4, 5	4, 5	5, 5	5, 5	36, 38	5, 5	5, 5	9, 10	45, 48
	ICC	Mean	0.58	0.59	0.60	0.60	0.54	0.77	0.71	0.31	0.51	0.61	0.51	0.56	0.54
		95% CI	0.45, 0.69	0.46, 0.70	0.47, 0.70	0.46, 0.70	0.39, 0.65	0.70, 0.83	0.62, 0.78	0.10, 0.48	0.35, 0.64	0.48, 0.71	0.36, 0.63	0.42, 0.67	0.36, 0.66
Ground Truth	Score	Median	5	5	5	5	5	5	5	5	39	5	5	10	48
		IQR	4, 5	5, 5	4, 5	5, 5	5, 5	5, 5	5, 5	5, 5	37, 39	5, 5	5, 5	10, 10	47, 49
	ICC	Mean	0.57	0.04	0.39	0.56	0.42	0.61	0.55	0.52	0.48	0.65	0.40	0.57	0.54
		95% CI	0.36, 0.70	0.25, 0.27	0.21, 0.54	0.42, 0.67	0.24, 0.56	0.49, 0.71	0.41, 0.66	0.36, 0.64	0.27, 0.63	0.54, 0.74	0.22, 0.55	0.44, 0.68	0.34, 0.67
Score between two maskings		*p*-value	<0.001 *	0.25	<0.001 *	<0.001 *	<0.001 *	<0.001 *	<0.001 *	0.39	<0.001 *	<0.001 *	<0.001 *	<0.001 *	<0.001 *

IQR, interquartile range; ICC, intraclass correlation coefficient; Tm, trapezium; Td, trapezoid; C, capitate; H, hamate; P, pisiform; Tr, triquetrum; L, lunate; S, scaphoid; R, distal radius; U, distal ulna. The Wilcoxon signed rank test was used to compare the Turing test results between the prediction and the ground truth masking. * *p*-values < 0.05 were considered statistically significant. Values of ICC less than 0.5, between 0.5 and 0.75, between 0.75 and 0.9, and greater than 0.90 were indicative of poor, moderate, good, and excellent reliability, respectively.

4. Discussion

In this study, we have proposed a Fine Mask R-CNN, and this model performed better, with a 0.95 (0.01) Dice coefficient for the segmentation of ten wrist bones, including eight carpal bones and two distal forearm bones, from wrist radiographs of people between 18 and 80 years old. Currently, there are two established neural network models specifically used for image segmentation in the computer imaging field: the fully convolutional neural network (FCN) and Mask R-CNN. Meng et al. reported that FCN could segment the carpal site with a Dice coefficient of 0.78 (0.06), using hand and wrist radiographs of people between 0 and 18 years old [36]. Su et al. reported that carpal bones were successfully detected with a high Dice coefficient of 0.976 using threshold processing and boundary detection on hand radiograph images. However, this was only tested on 30 representative images of non-overlapping carpal bones [37].

We have assessed the performance of two approaches to the segmentation of ten wrist bones. Faisal et al. found that the range of Dice coefficients for the segmentation of eight carpal bones was 0.83~0.94 when the locally weighted K-means variational level set was applied, whereas the range was 0.91~0.96 when Fine Mask R-CNN was employed in our study [22]. Goo et al. showed that the mean Dice coefficient of the automatic segmentation of the distal ulna and radius with dynamic programing was about 0.90, when using forearm radiographs [17], while we achieved a mean [SD] Dice of 0.96 (0.01) with Fine Mask R-CNN. The use of a fracture detection CNN without segmentation, based on a Dense-161, for distal radio-ulnar fractures on plain radiographs showed a sensitivity of 90.3%, with a specificity of 90.3% [38]. The sensitivity and specificity of the CNN without segmentation in terms of detecting distal radial fractures (using EfcientNet-B2 in frontal view and EfcientNet-B4 in lateral view wrist radiographs) were 98.7% and 100%, respectively [39]. The use of a segmentation and fracture detection CNN, based on a DenseNet-121, for the automated detection of scaphoid fractures on plain radiographs achieved a Dice coefficient of 0.974 (0.014) and a sensitivity of 78%, with a specificity of 84%. This network could achieve performance levels comparable to human observation in detecting scaphoid fractures on radiographs [11]. Our proposed network for the segmentation of ten wrist bones could assist in the automatic detection of various wrist bone fractures on wrist radiographs.

Most studies on wrist bone segmentation have used the wrist radiographs of young children. Wrist bones are formed during infancy, and increasingly overlap as their size increases [13,37,40]. In our study using Fine Mask R-CNN on adults' wrist radiographs, the performance for scaphoid, capitate, hamate, and lunate bones achieved Dice coefficients of over 0.95, because these bones are relatively large, and the overlap area with other bones is relatively small. However, the Dice values of some were lower, such as 0.93 for the trapezium, 0.91 for the trapezoid, and 0.93 for the pisiform. This is because the trapezium and trapezoid overlap in almost all areas in men over 7 years of age and women over 5 years of age [13], and the trapezium, trapezoid, and pisiform wrist bones overlap on the wrist PA radiographs of adults [41]. We have proposed a two-stage method that extracts the ROI from a wrist X-ray image first, and then segments the 10 bones within to solve this problem. Additionally, in the segmentation module based on Mask R-CNN, using an encoder–decoder-type network, spatial information can be preserved. This helped us to improve the segmentation performance by using the preserved spatial information. However, the capacity for the delineation of overlapping bones, such as the trapezium, trapezoid, and pisiform, was still worse than the others.

The Turing test is an important measure of how "intelligent" a deep learning model is. In a study on the automatic segmentation of a clinical target volume in rectal cancer patients, at least three out of ten clinicians thought that the predicted masking in this region was better than the ground truth masking [42]. This is the first study to carry out a Turing test on the automatic segmentation of ten wrist bones using wrist radiographs. The evaluators could not assign superiority between the masking predicted by our network and the ground truth masking performed by clinicians for the segmentation of two (trapezoid and scaphoid) wrist bones

Several limitations of this study should be considered. First, the data on the wrist radiographs and the patients originated from a single center, and our proposed model might not be suitable for other hospitals. Second, our proposed method was not an end-to-end network. Since Fine Mask R-CNN consists of two different neural networks—wrist ROI detection and wrist segmentation networks, the gradient cannot be shared directly between them. Therefore, our work needs to be extended to assess end-to-end networks that will establish a trainable attention module for future work. Finally, bias could not be eliminated from the Turing test because the test was performed by three radiologists from one center, without double blindness or randomization.

5. Conclusions

Our proposed CNN model exhibited a highly favorable performance in the automatic segmentation of ten overlapping wrist bones, consisting of eight carpal bones and the distal ulna and radius carpal bones, on plain wrist radiographs.

Author Contributions: J.O. and J.L. (Jongwoo Lim) conceived the study and designed the trial. J.O., B.-k.K., Y.H., M.S.Y. and J.L. (Juncheol Lee) supervised the trial and were involved in data collection; Y.H., J.R., B.-k.K. and J.L. (Jongwoo Lim) analyzed all images and data; Y.H., B.-K.K., J.L. (Jongwoo Lim) and J.O. drafted the manuscript, and B.-k.K., Y.H., J.O., J.L. (Jongwoo Lim), J.R., M.S.Y., J.L. (Juncheol Lee) and S.R. substantially contributed to its revision; J.O. and J.L. (Jongwoo Lim) take responsibility for the content of the paper. All authors have read and agreed to the published version of the manuscript.

Funding: This study was supported by the National Research Foundation of Korea (NRF-2022R1A2C-1012627) and by Institute of Information & communications Technology Planning & Evaluation (IITP) grant funded by the Korea government (MSIT) (No.2020-0-01373, Artificial Intelligence Graduate School Program (Hanyang University)).

Institutional Review Board Statement: The study was conducted in accordance with the Declaration of Helsinki, and approved by the Institutional Review Board of Hanyang University Hospital (HYUH 2020-03-037).

Informed Consent Statement: Informed consent was waived by the IRB due to the retrospective study.

Data Availability Statement: The data presented in this study are available on request from the corresponding author.

Conflicts of Interest: The authors declare no conflict of interest.

Abbreviations

CNN	convolution neural network
PA	Posteroanterior
AP	Anteroposterior
PACS	picture archiving and communication system
ROI	region of interest
SSD	Single-Shot Multibox Detector
SGD	stochastic gradient descent
Dice	Dice coefficient
IQR	interquartile ranges
SD	standard deviation
ICC	intraclass correlation coefficient

References

1. Larsen, C.F.; Lauritsen, J. Epidemiology of acute wrist trauma. *Int. J. Epidemiol.* **1993**, *22*, 911–916. [CrossRef] [PubMed]
2. Ferguson, R.; Riley, N.D.; Wijendra, A.; Thurley, N.; Carr, A.J.; Bjf, D. Wrist pain: A systematic review of prevalence and risk factors-What is the role of occupation and activity? *BMC Musculoskelet. Disord.* **2019**, *20*, 542. [CrossRef] [PubMed]
3. Linn, M.R.; Mann, F.A.; Gilula, L.A. Imaging the symptomatic wrist. *Orthop. Clin. N. Am.* **1990**, *21*, 515–543. [CrossRef]

4. Lee, R.K.; Griffith, J.F.; Ng, A.W.; Wong, C.W. Imaging of radial wrist pain. I. Imaging modalities and anatomy. *Skelet. Radiol.* **2014**, *43*, 713–724. [CrossRef] [PubMed]
5. Porteous, R.; Harish, S.; Parasu, N. Imaging of ulnar-sided wrist pain. *Can. Assoc. Radiol. J.* **2012**, *63*, 18–29. [CrossRef]
6. Bhat, A.K.; Kumar, B.; Acharya, A. Radiographic imaging of the wrist. *Indian J. Plast. Surg.* **2011**, *44*, 186–196. [CrossRef]
7. Hemke, R.; Buckless, C.G.; Tsao, A.; Wang, B.; Torriani, M. Deep learning for automated segmentation of pelvic muscles, fat, and bone from CT studies for body composition assessment. *Skelet. Radiol.* **2020**, *49*, 387–395. [CrossRef]
8. Rehman, F.; Shah, S.I.A.; Riaz, M.N.; Gilani, S.O. A region-based deep level set formulation for vertebral bone segmentation of osteoporotic fractures. *J. Digit. Imaging* **2020**, *33*, 191–203. [CrossRef]
9. Peng, L.-Q.; Guo, Y.-C.; Wan, L.; Liu, T.-A.; Wang, P.; Zhao, H.; Wang, Y.-H. Forensic bone age estimation of adolescent pelvis X-rays based on two-stage convolutional neural network. *Int. J. Leg. Med.* **2022**, *136*, 797–810. [CrossRef]
10. Foster, B.; Joshi, A.; Borgese, M.; Abdelhafez, Y.; Boutin, R.D.; Chaudhari, A.J. WRIST: A WRist Image Segmentation Toolkit for carpal bone delineation from MRI. *Comput. Med. Imaging Graph.* **2018**, *63*, 31–40. [CrossRef]
11. Hendrix, N.; Scholten, E.; Vernhout, B.; Bruijnen, G.; Maresch, B.; de Jong, M.; Diepstraten, S.; Bollen, S.; Schalekamp, S.; de Rooij, M.; et al. Development and Validation of a Convolutional Neural Network for Automated Detection of Scaphoid Fractures on Conventional Radiographs. *Radiol. Artif. Intell.* **2021**, *3*, e200260. [CrossRef] [PubMed]
12. Manos, G.; Cairns, A.; Ricketts, I.; Sinclair, D. Automatic segmentation of hand-wrist radiographs. *Image Vis. Comput.* **1993**, *11*, 100–111. [CrossRef]
13. Zhang, A.; Gertych, A.; Liu, B.J. Automatic bone age assessment for young children from newborn to 7-year-old using carpal bones. *Comput. Med. Imaging Graph.* **2007**, *31*, 299–310. [CrossRef] [PubMed]
14. Włodarczyk, J.; Czaplicka, K.; Tabor, Z.; Wojciechowski, W.; Urbanik, A. Segmentation of bones in magnetic resonance images of the wrist. *Int. J. Comput. Assist. Radiol. Surg.* **2015**, *10*, 419–431. [CrossRef]
15. Włodarczyk, J.; Wojciechowski, W.; Czaplicka, K.; Urbanik, A.; Tabor, Z. Fast automated segmentation of wrist bones in magnetic resonance images. *Comput. Biol. Med.* **2015**, *65*, 44–53. [CrossRef]
16. Koch, M.; Schwing, A.G.; Comaniciu, D.; Pollefeys, M. Fully automatic segmentation of wrist bones for arthritis patients. In Proceedings of the 2011 IEEE International Symposium on Biomedical Imaging: From Nano to Macro, Chicago, IL, USA, 30 March–2 April 2011; pp. 636–640.
17. Gou, X.; Rao, Y.; Feng, X.; Yun, Z.; Yang, W. Automatic Segmentation of Ulna and Radius in Forearm Radiographs. *Comput. Math Methods Med.* **2019**, *2019*, 6490161. [CrossRef]
18. Manos, G.K.; Cairns, A.Y.; Rickets, I.W.; Sinclair, D. Segmenting radiographs of the hand and wrist. *Comput. Methods Programs Biomed.* **1994**, *43*, 227–237. [CrossRef]
19. Canny, J. A computational approach to edge detection. *IEEE Trans. Pattern Anal. Mach. Intell.* **1986**, *6*, 679–698. [CrossRef]
20. Li, J.; Nebelung, S.; Schock, J.; Rath, B.; Tingart, M.; Liu, Y.; Siroros, N.; Eschweiler, J. A Novel Combined Level Set Model for Carpus Segmentation from Magnetic Resonance Images with Prior Knowledge aligned in Polar Coordinate System. *Comput. Methods Programs Biomed.* **2021**, *208*, 106245. [CrossRef]
21. Sebastian, T.B.; Tek, H.; Crisco, J.J.; Kimia, B.B. Segmentation of carpal bones from CT images using skeletally coupled deformable models. *Med. Image Anal.* **2003**, *7*, 21–45. [CrossRef]
22. Faisal, A.; Khalil, A.; Chai, H.Y.; Lai, K.W. X-ray carpal bone segmentation and area measurement. *Multimed. Tools Appl.* **2021**, 1–12. [CrossRef]
23. Giordano, D.; Spampinato, C.; Scarciofalo, G.; Leonardi, R. An automatic system for skeletal bone age measurement by robust processing of carpal and epiphysial/metaphysial bones. *IEEE Trans. Instrum. Meas.* **2010**, *59*, 2539–2553. [CrossRef]
24. He, K.; Gkioxari, G.; Dollár, P.; Girshick, R. Mask r-cnn. In Proceedings of the IEEE International Conference on Computer Vision, Venice, Italy, 22–29 October 2017; pp. 2961–2969.
25. Kwon, G.; Ryu, J.; Oh, J.; Lim, J.; Kang, B.-K.; Ahn, C.; Bae, J.; Lee, D.K. Deep learning algorithms for detecting and visualising intussusception on plain abdominal radiography in children: A retrospective multicenter study. *Sci. Rep.* **2020**, *10*, 17582. [CrossRef] [PubMed]
26. Guan, Q.; Huang, Y.; Zhong, Z.; Zheng, Z.; Zheng, L.; Yang, Y. Diagnose like a radiologist: Attention guided convolutional neural network for thorax disease classification. *arXiv* **2018**, arXiv:1801.09927.
27. Liu, W.; Anguelov, D.; Erhan, D.; Szegedy, C.; Reed, S.; Fu, C.Y.; Berg, A.C. SSD: Single-Shot Multibox Detector. In *European Conference on Computer Vision*; Springer: Cham, Switzerland, 2016. [CrossRef]
28. Alsinan, A.Z.; Patel, V.M.; Hacihaliloglu, I. Automatic segmentation of bone surfaces from ultrasound using a filter-layer-guided CNN. *Int. J. Comput. Assist. Radiol. Surg.* **2019**, *14*, 775–783. [CrossRef] [PubMed]
29. Chen, L.; Zhou, X.; Wang, M.; Qiu, J.; Cao, M.; Mao, K. ARU-Net: Research and Application for Wrist Reference Bone Segmentation. In Proceedings of the 2019 International Conference on Wireless and Mobile Computing, Networking and Communications (WiMob), Barcelona, Spain, 21–23 October 2019; pp. 1–5.
30. Nakatsu, K.; Rahman, R.; Morita, K.; Fujita, D.; Kobashi, S. Automatic Carpal Site Detection Method for Evaluation of Rheumatoid Arthritis Using Deep Learning. *J. Adv. Comput. Intell. Intell. Inform.* **2022**, *26*, 42–50. [CrossRef]
31. Ronneberger, O.; Philipp, F.; Thomas, B. U-net: Convolutional networks for biomedical image segmentation. In *International Conference on Medical Image Computing and Computer-Assisted Intervention*; Springer: Cham, Switzerland, 2015; pp. 234–241.

32. Kirillov, A.; Wu, Y.; He, K.; Girshick, R. Pointrend: Image segmentation as rendering. In Proceedings of the IEEE/CVF Conference on Computer Vision and Pattern Recognition, Online, 14–19 June 2020; pp. 9799–9808.
33. Frid-Adar, M.; Ben-Cohen, A.; Amer, R.; Greenspan, H. Improving the Segmentation of Anatomical Structures in Chest Radiographs Using U-Net with an ImageNet Pre-Trained Encoder. In *Image Analysis for Moving Organ, Breast, and Thoracic Images*; Springer: Cham, Switzerland, 2018; Volume 11040, pp. 159–168. [CrossRef]
34. Punn, N.S.; Agarwal, S. Automated Diagnosis of COVID-19 with Limited Posteroanterior Chest X-Ray Images Using Fine-Tuned Deep Neural Networks. *Appl. Intell.* 2021, *51*, 2689–2702. [CrossRef]
35. Koo, T.K.; Li, M.Y. A guideline of selecting and reporting intraclass correlation coefficients for reliability research. *J. Chiropr. Med.* 2016, *15*, 155–163. [CrossRef]
36. Meng, L.K.; Khalil, A.; Nizar, M.H.A.; Nisham, M.K.; Pingguan-Murphy, B.; Hum, Y.C.; Salim, M.I.M.; Lai, K.W. Carpal bone segmentation using fully convolutional neural network. *Curr. Med. Imaging Rev.* 2019, *15*, 983–989. [CrossRef]
37. Su, L.; Fu, X.; Zhang, X.; Cheng, X.; Ma, Y.; Gan, Y.; Hu, Q. Delineation of Carpal Bones From Hand X-Ray Images Through Prior Model, and Integration of Region-Based and Boundary-Based Segmentations. *IEEE Access* 2018, *6*, 19993–20008. [CrossRef]
38. Kim, M.W.; Jung, J.; Park, S.J.; Park, Y.S.; Yi, J.H.; Yang, W.S.; Kim, J.H.; Cho, B.J.; Ha, S.O. Application of convolutional neural networks for distal radio-ulnar fracture detection on plain radiographs in the emergency room. *Clin. Exp. Emerg. Med.* 2021, *8*, 120–127. [CrossRef] [PubMed]
39. Suzuki, T.; Maki, S.; Yamazaki, T.; Wakita, H.; Toguchi, Y.; Horii, M.; Yamauchi, T.; Kawamura, K.; Aramomi, M.; Sugiyama, H.; et al. Detecting Distal Radial Fractures from Wrist Radiographs Using a Deep Convolutional Neural Network with an Accuracy Comparable to Hand Orthopedic Surgeons. *J. Digit. Imaging* 2022, *35*, 39–46. [CrossRef] [PubMed]
40. Somkantha, K.; Theera-Umpon, N.; Auephanwiriyakul, S. Bone age assessment in young children using automatic carpal bone feature extraction and support vector regression. *J. Digit. Imaging* 2011, *24*, 1044–1058. [CrossRef]
41. Gilula, L.A. Carpal injuries: Analytical approach and case exercises. *AJR Am. J. Roentgenol.* 1979, *133*, 513–517. [CrossRef] [PubMed]
42. Wu, Y.; Kang, K.; Han, C.; Wang, S.; Chen, Q.; Chen, Y.; Zhang, F.; Liu, Z. A blind randomized validated convolutional neural network for auto-segmentation of clinical target volume in rectal cancer patients receiving neoadjuvant radiotherapy. *Cancer Med.* 2022, *11*, 166–175. [CrossRef]

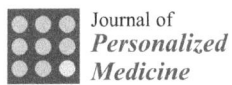

Article

Management of Displaced Midshaft Clavicle Fractures with Figure-of-Eight Bandage: The Impact of Residual Shortening on Shoulder Function

Carlo Biz [1], Davide Scucchiari [1], Assunta Pozzuoli [1,2,*], Elisa Belluzzi [1,2], Nicola Luigi Bragazzi [3], Antonio Berizzi [1,*] and Pietro Ruggieri [1]

[1] Orthopedics and Orthopedic Oncology, Department of Surgery, Oncology and Gastroenterology DiSCOG, University of Padova, Via Giustiniani 3, 35128 Padova, Italy; carlo.biz@unipd.it (C.B.); davide.scucchiari@gmail.com (D.S.); elisa.belluzzi@unipd.it (E.B.); pietro.ruggieri@unipd.it (P.R.)

[2] Musculoskeletal Pathology and Oncology Laboratory, Department of Surgery, Oncology and Gastroenterology, University of Padova, Via Giustiniani 3, 35128 Padova, Italy

[3] Laboratory for Industrial and Applied Mathematics (LIAM), Department of Mathematics and Statistics, York University, Toronto, ON M3J 1P3, Canada; robertobragazzi@gmail.com

* Correspondence: assunta.pozzuoli@unipd.it (A.P.); antonio.berizzi@unipd.it (A.B.); Tel.: +39-049-821-3348 (A.P.); +39-049-821-3310 (A.B.)

Abstract: The treatment of displaced midshaft clavicle fractures (MCFs) is still controversial. The aims of our study were to evaluate clinical and radiological outcomes and complications of patients with displaced MCFs managed nonoperatively and to identify potential predictive factors of worse clinical outcomes. Seventy-five patients with displaced MCFs were enrolled and treated nonoperatively with a figure-of-eight bandage (F8-B). Initial shortening (IS) and displacement (ID) of fragments were radiographically evaluated at the time of diagnosis and immediately after F8-B application by residual shortening (RS) and displacement (RD). The clavicle shortening ratio was evaluated clinically at last follow-up. Functional outcomes were assessed using Constant (CS), q-DASH, DASH work and DASH sport scores. Cosmetic outcomes and rate of complications were evaluated. Good to very good mid-term clinical results were achieved by using the institutional treatment protocol. Multiple regression identified RS as an independent predictor of shoulder function, while RD affects fracture healing. These findings support the efficacy of our institutional protocol and thus could be useful for orthopedic surgeons during the decision-making process.

Keywords: clavicle fracture; midshaft fractures; displaced fractures; conservative treatment

1. Introduction

Clavicle fractures represent 2.6–4% of all fractures on average [1], and up to 82% of them affect the clavicle midshaft [2]. A male predominance is reported, accounting for about 70% in young active male patients, while females are slightly more affected in elderly age [1,3,4]. These injuries commonly occur during athletic or recreational activities as the result of an axial force caused by a fall on the shoulder or on an outstretched hand, and traffic accidents or, less often, by a direct hit to the shoulder [5]. Midshaft clavicle fractures (MCFs) are among the most common upper extremity injuries managed by orthopedic trauma surgeons, and it is estimated that about half of all MCFs are displaced [6].

Clinical manifestations of clavicle fractures usually include pain and visible bone deformity as a consequence of the displacement of clavicle fragments [4].

Non-displaced MCFs are satisfactorily treated nonoperatively by sling immobilization, while the treatment of displaced fractures, which are the most frequent, is still under debate [7].

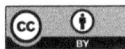

Acute displaced MCFs are traditionally managed successfully nonoperatively [8] showing good to very good results [3,9], while surgery becomes the treatment of choice in cases of failure of conservative treatment [10,11].

However, recent studies reporting higher nonunion rates after nonoperative treatment and an allegedly better clinical outcome after operative treatment, have led to a shift from nonoperative to operative treatment in the last 15–20 years [12–14]. Surgically treated patients, however, end up having to undergo second surgery for device removal procedures in more than 85% of cases [15].

To date, there are few absolute indications for early surgical fixation. Surgery is recommended in cases of open fractures, neurological deficiencies, compromised skin conditions, vascular injury, ipsilateral serial rib fractures, floating shoulder, widely displaced and comminuted fractures [8,16].

Nevertheless, current studies, including recent randomized controlled trials and meta-analyses, are still conflicting and fail to demonstrate the absolute superiority of surgical versus conservative management [6,14,17–20]. Several studies report better outcomes of surgery along with lower risk of nonunion compared to nonoperative management [18,21]. Conversely, other studies do not show differences in functional outcomes between conservative treatment and plate fixation of acute displaced MCFs, not only at one year of follow-up [10,13,14,22–26], but also after 24 weeks as well as after five years of follow-up [27]. Furthermore, surgical fixation is associated with complications in up to 29% of patients, such as wound infections, neurologic symptoms, frozen shoulder and implant-related problems [12].

Importantly, the identification of predictive factors of worse clinical outcome or nonunion or symptomatic malunion is of great interest for the orthopedic surgeons as it would enable the identification of those patients at high risk of conservative treatment failure and help to avoid surgery overtreatment [28]. Jørgensen et al. published a systematic review reporting displacement as a likely risk factor of nonunion, while smoking, fracture comminution, age, gender and shortening were defined as doubtfully nonunion risk factors [28].

In a previous study published by our research group, predictive factors of delayed union and nonunion in adult patients with an MCF treated with a figure-of-eight bandage (F8-B) were investigated [29]. A residual displacement (RD) of 104%, assessed immediately after the application of the F8-B, was found to be a predictor that can help to differentiate patients who will heal, from patients who will develop delayed union and nonunion. Moreover, an RD of 140% was identified as an optimal cut-off point to distinguish between delayed union and nonunion [29]. Based on these findings, a treatment protocol for displaced MCFs was adopted in our clinic.

The objectives of this single-center study were (1) to evaluate clinical and radiological outcomes of patients with displaced MCFs managed nonoperatively following our institutional protocol and (2) to identify potential predictive factors of worse clinical outcomes.

2. Materials and Methods

2.1. Patient Selection

This study was designed as a single-center, retrospective, non-comparative case series, including patients affected by a displaced MCF between December 2015 and December 2018 and treated nonoperatively with an F8-B. All subjects participating in this experimental study received a thorough explanation of the risks and benefits of inclusion and gave their written informed consent to publish the data. This study was approved by the Institutional Ethics Committee (CESC code 189N/AO/21) and was performed in accordance with the ethical standards of the 1964 Declaration of Helsinki as revised in 2000 and those of Good Clinical Practice [30].

Inclusion criteria were: (1) patients with a traumatic, non-pathological, acute displaced MCF; (2) active patients between 18 and 65 years old; (3) at least 1-year clinical and radiographic follow-up; (4) RD $\leq$ 140% (see Section 2.3. Patient assessment) [29]. Exclusion criteria were: (1) ipsilateral neurological involvement; (2) patients receiving chemotherapy, radiotherapy and/or immunotherapy; (3) patients with a bilateral clavicle fracture; (4) patients with previous injury or surgery of the ipsilateral clavicle and/or shoulder; (5) patients who did not complete the entire follow-up program; (6) competitive athletes; (7) polytrauma patients; (8) RD > 140% (see Section 2.3. Patient assessment).

2.2. Treatment Protocol

At our level-1 healthcare trauma center, a 1572-bed multi-disciplinary and multi-specialty regional university hospital, a highly standardized institutional treatment protocol, specific for patients with MCFs, was adopted (Figure 1).

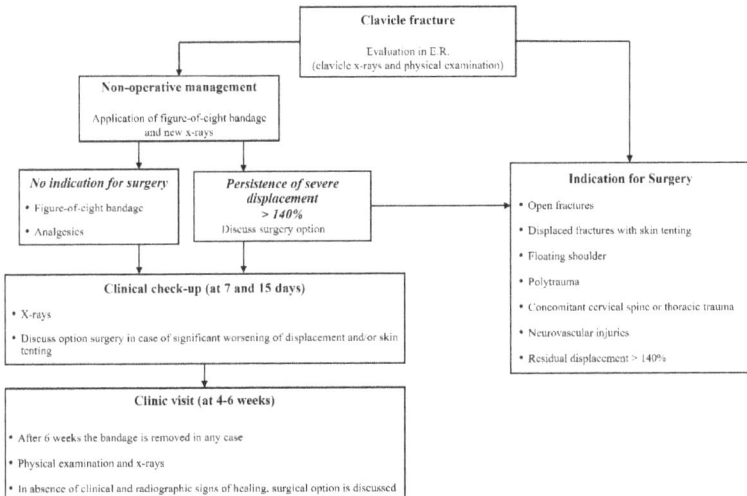

Figure 1. Institutional treatment protocol for displaced midshaft clavicle fracture of adult patients.

Patients were first evaluated by a trauma surgeon from our unit at the Emergency Room (ER) with plain X-rays (standard anteroposterior and 20° cephalic tilt views) (Figure 2: clinical case).

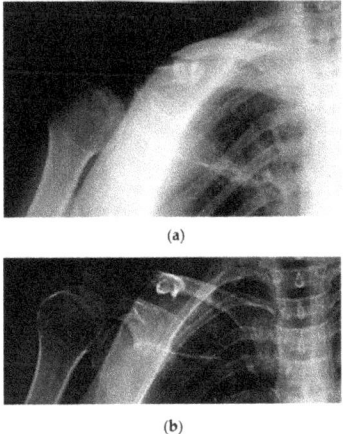

Figure 2. Radiographic images showing a traumatic displaced midshaft fracture of the right (dominant) clavicle in a 53-year-old female patient: (**a**) Cephalic tilt and; (**b**) anteroposterior X-ray views.

A careful physical examination was performed to evaluate functional impairment of the shoulder but also of the whole upper limb to exclude rare but possible associated injuries involving the brachial plexus or the subclavian vessels [4,16,31,32].

Other rare but potentially serious complications could involve the chest, such as the pneumothorax or hemothorax, which can be excluded with both thorough clinical and radiographic assessments [4,33–38].

Patients were referred to surgery in case of open fractures, displaced fractures with skin tenting, "floating shoulder", polytrauma, concomitant cervical spine or thoracic trauma and neurovascular injuries. In all other cases, nonoperative management with an F8-B was suggested. Standard X-rays were repeated immediately after F8-B application in the ER to check the alignment of the fragments. Patients received thorough instructions on correct bandage use and positioning to avoid both decubitus ulcers in the axillary region and compression of the neurovascular bundle. All active movements of the shoulder were limited by the application of the F8-B; passive range of motion not above 90° forward flexion was permitted, while slight movements of the hand and the elbow (without load) were encouraged to prevent joint contractures and edema [3].

When severe RD persisted (>140%) after F8-B application, or when mechanical factors like soft tissue interposition, comminution or vertical fragments that impair reduction were suspected, surgical intervention was proposed [28].

Nonoperatively treated patients underwent both clinical and radiographic assessments at 7 days and 14 days after trauma to evaluate bandage tolerability and position and any possible worsening of fractures. When there was significant worsening of displacement and/or skin tenting, the option of surgery was discussed with the patient. The F8-B was maintained for 4–6 weeks, depending on fracture healing.

In case of the absence of clinical and radiographic signs of healing after 6 weeks, including CT scan evaluation, the bandage was removed, and surgical reconstruction was discussed with the patient (Figure 3: clinical case).

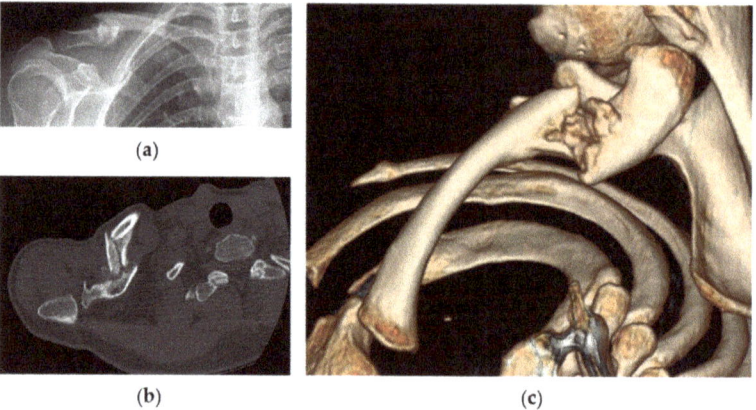

Figure 3. Radiographic images of the same patient showing right clavicle nonunion at 4-month follow-up: (**a**) anteroposterior X-ray view of the clavicle; (**b**) axial CT-scan evaluation of nonunion and; (**c**) 3D reconstruction.

2.3. Patient Assessment

Data collection was retrospectively performed by external and independent investigators, not involved in the patients' treatment. Age, gender, body mass index (BMI), smoking status, presence of hypercholesterolemia and/or hypertension, mechanism of trauma, affected side and dominant limb involvement were recorded as baseline characteristics of the cohort.

Based on standard X-rays performed at patient admission at the ER of our hospital, radiographic fracture features were recorded as follows: fracture type (FT) according to the AO/OTA (Association for Osteosynthesis/Orthopedic Trauma Association) Classification [24]; initial shortening (IS) and residual shortening (RS), defined as the overlap of proximal and distal fragments and assessed as a percentage of the same clavicle length on a standard antero-posterior view, measured before and after the F8-B application; initial displacement (ID) and residual displacement (RD), measured as a percentage of the clavicle width at the fracture site on a 20° cephalic tilt view of the clavicle before and after the F8-B [29].

Clinical follow-up was performed on a weekly basis for two weeks after trauma and afterwards at 1-, 3-, 6-, and 12-months post-injury, while radiographic follow-up was prolonged until fracture union.

At the last follow-up visit, about one year after trauma, functional outcomes were measured by the Constant–Murley Score (CS) [25] and the Quick Disability of the Arm, Shoulder and Hand score (qDASH) [26]. CS consists of four items: pain; activities of daily living (ADL); range of motion (ROM); and strength. CS ranges from 0 to 100, indicating worst to optimum shoulder function. The qDASH score ranges from 0 to 100 with the latter representing the most disability and dysfunction; the optional qDASH work and sport modules were also used.

In addition, time of return to work and return to sport or recreational activities were evaluated. A visual analogue scale (VAS) (range 0–10) was adopted to assess patient satisfaction of their functional status. The cosmetic outcome was assessed as a patient-reported outcome measure, asking patients if the treatment received had resulted in any negative effect on their quality of life.

The final clavicle shortening ratio compared with the contralateral clavicle was also assessed with a measuring tape at the last follow-up.

Finally, any complications were also recorded.

2.4. Nonoperative Rehabilitation Protocol

The F8-B was removed at 4–6 weeks. Then, the patients were trained to perform Codman exercises [39] and gradually, active shoulder movements as much as could be tolerated to achieve a full range of motion (ROM) over the next 3 or 4 weeks.

Lifting weight, heavy physical activity and contact sports were allowed only after complete clinical-radiological union of the fracture.

2.5. Statistical Analysis

Categorical variables were computed as percentages, while continuous parameters were expressed as means ± standard deviations. Normality of the data distribution was checked by means of a Shapiro–Wilk test. Univariate analyses were conducted using Student's t-test and analysis of variance (ANOVA). Correlational analysis was conducted to shed light on the nature of the association between the various variables under study using the correlation coefficient assessment or its parametric version, depending on the normality of data distribution. Multivariate analysis of covariance (MANCOVA) was performed to identify the predictors of the outcome variables [40]. Partial eta squared was computed as effect size. MANCOVA assumptions (normal distribution of the dependent variables within groups; homogeneity of variance for each dependent variable and homogeneity of covariance for all the levels of the independent variable; linear relationship between the dependent variable and the covariates) were checked and met.

In case of statistical significance of a parameter, receiver operating characteristics (ROC) analysis was performed to quantitatively assess the effectiveness of a given classifier in terms of sensitivity and specificity. ROC analysis enables computing discrimination thresholds for variables of interest. We conducted ROC analysis by calculating the area under the curve (AUC) to obtain specific cut-off values. More specifically, the Youden J index was computed to identify the most acceptable trade-off in terms of sensitivity and specificity.

For all statistical analyses, a p-value less than 0.05 was considered statistically significant. All statistical analyses were carried out by means of the commercial software "Statistical Package for the Social Sciences" (SPSS, version 28.0 for Windows, IBM Corporation, Armonk, NY, USA) by an independent statistician.

3. Results

Seventy-five patients treated nonoperatively met the inclusion criteria and were enrolled in the study.

Demographic and clinical characteristics of the patients are reported in Table 1.

Table 1. Demographic and clinical characteristics of overall patients.

Variable	Patients Enrolled $n = 75$
Age, mean (SD)	42.8 (13.7)
Gender, number (%)	
male	62 (82.7)
female	13 (17.3)
BMI, mean (SD)	24.1 (2.3)
Smoking status, number (%)	
active	33 (44.0)
inactive	42 (56.0)
Hypercholesterolemia, number (%)	
LDL $\geq$ 240 mg/dL	7 (9.3)
LDL < 240 md/dL	68 (90.7)
Hypertension, number (%)	
Systolic $\geq$ 130, Diastolic $\geq$ 80	17 (22.7)
Systolic < 130, Diastolic < 80	58 (77.3)
Type of trauma, number (%)	
Bike Fall	29 (38.7)
Motorcycle trauma	21 (28.0)
Sport injury	16 (21.3)
Simple fall	9 (12.0)
Dominant side involved, number (%)	31 (41.3)

SD = Standard Deviation; BMI = Body Mass Index; LDL = Low Density Lipoproteins. (Hypercholesterolemia: LDL $\geq$ 240 mg/dL).

Mechanisms of trauma were a bike fall for twenty-nine cases (38.7%), a motorcycle trauma for twenty-one cases (28.0%), low energy traumas such as a sports injury for sixteen patients (21.3%) and a simple fall in nine patients (12.0%).

The radiographic parameters of enrolled patients are reported in Table 2.

The mean IS and RS were 5.4 ± 4.6% and 3.4 ± 3.6%, while mean ID and RD were 113 ± 43.4% and 91.8 ± 30.8 %, respectively. Mean follow-up time was 27.5 ± 7.5 months.

A mean total CS of 96.8 ± 5.6 and total qDASH of 4.2 ± 6.3 were recorded (Table 3).

Mean time of return to work was 2.5 ± 1.1 months, while mean time of return to sports or recreational activities was 4.1 ± 1.8 months. Mean patient satisfaction was 7.6 ± 1.0. Thirty patients (40%) had cosmetic problems. The mean shortening ratio at last follow-up was 3.5 ± 3.5% (Table 3).

Regarding complications, refractures and delayed healing were reported in five and eleven patients, respectively.

All cases of refracture occurred in clinically and radiographically healed patients, after a forceful trauma, and at least four months after the first trauma. All cases were subsequently treated surgically. Conversely, delayed healing is referred to fractures not healed clinically and radiographically within three months from the trauma, but healed later within five months. The mean RD of delayed healed patients was 120.4% ± 15.8.

Table 2. Radiological characteristics of patients.

Variable	Patients Enrolled n = 75
Type of fracture, number (%)	
A1	5 (6.7)
A2	20 (26.7)
A3	6 (8.0)
B1	3 (4.0)
B2	13 (17.3)
B3	28 (37.3)
Initial shortening (%), mean (SD)	5.4 (4.6)
Residual shortening (%), mean (SD)	3.4 (3.6)
Initial displacement (%), mean (SD)	113 (43.4)
Residual displacement (%), mean (SD)	91.8 (30.8)

SD = Standard Deviation.

Table 3. Clinical outcomes of patients at follow-up (Mean follow-up time was 27.5 ± 7.5 months).

Outcomes	Patients Enrolled n = 75
Constant score, mean (SD)	
Total	96.8 (5.6)
Pain subscale	14.6 (1.2)
Activity Daily Living subscale	19.6 (1.2)
Range of movement subscale	39.3 (1.5)
Strength subscale	23.3 (3.1)
qDASH score, mean (SD)	
Total	4.2 (6.3)
Work	3.5 (9.1)
Sport	5.2 (11.8)
Return to work (months), mean (SD)	2.5 (1.1)
Return to sport (months), mean (SD)	4.1 (1.8)
VAS satisfaction, mean (SD)	7.6 (1.0)
Cosmetic problem, number (%)	30 (40)
Shortening ratio (%), mean (SD)	3.5 (3.5)

SD = Standard Deviation; qDASH = Quick Disabilities of the Arm, Shoulder and Hand; VAS = Visual Analogic Scale.

None of the patients suffered nonunion.

Correlations between clinical outcomes and radiological features were evaluated and reported in Table S1. Total CS and its subscales showed an inverse correlation with IS, RS and shortening ratio with higher values corresponding to lower total CS and subscale values. qDASH score, qDASH Work and qDASH sport correlated with IS, RS and shortening ratio, with higher values corresponding to greater qDASH values.

Return to work correlated in terms of ID, IS and shortening ratio with higher values corresponding to higher values of return to work.

No correlations were found between radiological features and return to sport.

Potential Predictive Factors

Multivariate analysis of covariance (MANCOVA) was performed to identify predictors of the outcome variables total CS and the qDASH score and their subscales. With the MANCOVA, RS resulted a statistically significant predictor (Table 4). All data of MANCOVA analysis are described in Table S2.

Table 4. Radiological predictors of shoulder function (MANCOVA).

Dependent Variable	Parameter	B	Std. Error	t	p-Value	95% Confidence Interval Lower Bound	95% Confidence Interval Upper Bound	Partial Eta Squared	Noncent. Parameter	Observed Power
CS total	Intercept	99.129	7.412	13.374	<.001	84.241	114.017	0.782	13.374	1.000
	ID	−0.020	0.017	−1.180	0.244	−0.054	0.014	0.027	1.180	0.212
	RD	0.016	0.025	0.637	0.527	−0.034	0.066	0.008	0.637	0.096
	IS	0.510	0.265	1.922	0.060	−0.023	1.042	0.069	1.922	0.470
	RS	−1.554	0.335	−4.637	**<0.001**	−2.228	−0.881	0.301	4.637	0.995
	Shortening ratio	−0.069	0.047	−1.461	0.150	−0.164	0.026	0.041	1.461	0.300
Pain	Intercept	10.282	2.068	4.972	<0.001	6.128	14.435	0.331	4.972	0.998
	ID	0.001	0.005	0.276	0.784	−0.008	0.011	0.002	0.276	0.058
	RD	0.008	0.007	1.079	0.286	−0.006	0.022	0.023	1.079	0.185
	IS	0.024	0.074	0.318	0.751	−0.125	0.172	0.002	0.318	0.061
	RS	−0.209	0.094	−2.235	**0.030**	−0.397	−0.021	0.091	2.235	0.592
	Shortening ratio	−0.004	0.013	−0.328	0.745	−0.031	0.022	0.002	0.328	0.062
ADL	Intercept	17.816	2.081	8.559	<0.001	13.635	21.997	0.594	8.559	1.000
	ID	−0.001	0.005	−0.315	0.754	−0.011	0.008	0.002	0.315	0.061
	RD	0.005	0.007	0.665	0.509	−0.009	0.019	0.009	0.665	0.100
	IS	0.048	0.074	0.647	0.521	−0.101	0.198	0.008	0.647	0.097
	RS	−0.193	0.094	−2.054	**0.045**	−0.382	−0.004	0.078	2.054	0.522
	Shortening ratio	−.032	0.013	−2.375	**0.021**	−0.058	−0.005	0.101	2.375	0.644
ROM	Intercept	45.954	2.442	18.816	<0.001	41.049	50.860	0.876	18.816	1.000
	ID	−0.006	0.006	−1.079	0.286	−0.017	0.005	0.023	1.079	0.185
	RD	−0.001	0.008	−.146	0.885	−0.018	0.015	0.000	0.146	0.052
	IS	0.095	0.087	1.090	0.281	−0.080	0.271	0.023	1.090	0.188
	RS	−0.272	0.110	−2.466	**0.017**	−0.494	−0.051	0.108	2.466	0.677
	Shortening ratio	−0.030	0.016	−1.905	0.063	−0.061	0.002	0.068	1.905	0.464
Strength	Intercept	25.679	4.299	5.974	<0.001	17.045	34.313	0.416	5.974	1.000
	ID	−0.015	0.010	−1.551	0.127	−0.035	0.004	0.046	1.551	0.331
	RD	0.006	0.015	0.397	0.693	−0.023	0.035	0.003	0.397	0.068
	IS	0.340	0.154	2.209	**0.032**	0.031	0.648	0.089	2.209	0.582
	RS	−0.799	0.194	−4.110	**<0.001**	−1.190	−0.409	0.253	4.110	0.981
	Shortening ratio	−.030	0.027	−1.082	0.284	−0.085	0.025	0.023	1.082	0.186

CS = Constant Score; ID = Initial Displacement; RD = Residual Displacement; IS = Initial Shortening; RS = Residual Shortening. Statistically significant p-value are bolded.

Age, BMI and smoking were not statistically significant predictors (data not shown).

An ROC curve analysis was performed to identify cut-off points for radiological features and functional outcomes.

RS (B coefficient = −1.55, $p < 0.001$; cut-off = 5, sensitivity 90.91%, specificity 45.16%) impacted total CS with lower RS values corresponding to higher total CS (Figure 4).

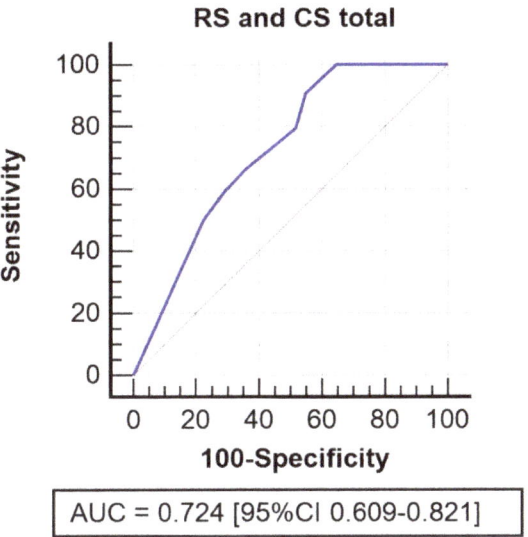

Figure 4. ROC curve. Receiver operating characteristic (ROC) curve for residual shortening and its impact on total CS.

RS impacted pain (B coefficient = −0.21, p = 0.030; cut-off = 5, sensitivity 87.10%, specificity 76.92%), with lower values of RS correlating with greater pain, as well as ROM (B coefficient = −0.27, p = 0.017; cut-off = 5, sensitivity 85.00%, specificity 60.00%) with a similar relationship, and ADL (B coefficient t = −0.19, p = 0.045; cut-off = 6, sensitivity 93.94%, specificity 77.78%), and in the latter case together with shortening ratio (B = −0.03, p = 0.021; cut-off = 6.7, sensitivity 95.45%, specificity 88.89%), with lower values of RS and shortening ratio corresponding to higher values of ADL.

RS (B coefficient = −0.80, p < 0.001; cut-off = 6, sensitivity 94.34%, specificity 36.36%) impacted strength. Lower RS values corresponded to greater strength values (Figure S1).

There was no significant determinant for qDASH, qDASH work and qDASH sport.

RS (B coefficient = 0.22, p = 0.012; cut-off = 2, sensitivity 59.32%, specificity 68.75%) impacted return to work, with higher RS values corresponding to later return to work.

4. Discussion

The objective of the present study was first to evaluate clinical and radiological outcomes of patients with displaced MCFs managed nonoperatively with an F8-B according to the protocol developed by our institution, which aimed to decrease nonunion rates, and secondly, to identify predictive factors of worse clinical outcomes. In our cohort, displaced MCFs mostly affected young male patients. Most of the patients were not overweight, had normal blood pressure and levels of LDL, all considered risk factors of developing nonunion [18,41–43]. Although almost 50% of patients were active smokers, smoking did not affect the functional outcomes evaluated in this study.

Most of the patients showed good clinical outcomes at their last follow-up appointment, both in terms of total CS and its subscales, and qDASH, qDASH work and qDASH sport.

In our study, according to Ziegler et al. [44] and Subramanyam et al. [18], who divided CS into four categories (very good 86–100, good 71–85, fair 56–70, poor <56), CS was very good in 93.3% of the patients and good in 6.7% of the patients, thus confirming the effective results of nonoperative management of displaced MCFs at medium-term follow-up [14,18,19].

These data were also supported by the good results of total qDASH (4.2 ± 6.3 points), DASH work (3.5 ± 9.1 points) and DASH sport (5.2 ± 11.8 points), highlighting the presence of low residual disability at follow-up as reported by Woltz et al., 2017 and Amer et al., 2020 [14,19].

Correlations between radiological features evaluated before and after the F8-B and clinical outcomes were also evaluated. More specifically, an inverse correlation was found between IS, RS and the shortening ratio and total CS and its subscales, confirming that lower values of shortening lead to higher values of CS, and therefore better functional outcomes.

These data were also confirmed with total qDASH, qDASH work and qDASH sport that directly correlate with IS, RS and shortening ratio with higher values of qDASH (higher upper limb disability) corresponding to higher values of shortening. Return to work was directly correlated with IS and RS, and the data obtained in our study are in line with what is reported in the recent literature [45].

VAS satisfaction showed good results with most of the patients satisfied. These data are similar to those of Woltz et al. (2018), even if some authors reported higher patient satisfaction in cases of early surgical management [46,47]. One of the most frequent reasons for patient dissatisfaction with the result of conservative treatment is poor cosmetic appearance, which emerged particularly among women [48]. Hence, cosmetic dissatisfaction was reported by 40% of our patients, a percentage lower than that reported in the literature [13].

Regarding complications, all the patients recovered with the conservative treatment and no nonunion was found, thus confirming the efficacy of the F8-B applied according to our institutional protocol, developed based on the findings of our previous analysis (including patients with RD $\leq$ 140%) [29]. This confirms the importance of fracture morphology with regard to healing.

Therefore, the absence of nonunion is an important result considering that the nonunion rate reported in the literature ranged between 5% and 20% after nonoperative treatment [19,20,42,49,50].

The 11 patients with delayed healing displayed an RD > 104% but less than 140%, in agreement with our previous study [29]. This result points out the importance not only of treatment selection but also of an appropriate follow-up of these patients that are at higher risk of having delayed healing with conservative treatment. In this context, our institutional protocol could be considered a useful guideline to identify how much displacement can be considered acceptable for nonoperative management (RD $\leq$ 140%), and when displaced fractures should be treated surgically.

Multivariate analysis was performed to identify predictive factors of worse clinical outcomes. RS results showed it to be a radiological predictor of worse shoulder function, as expressed by total CS with a cut-off value of five and its subscales: pain; ADL; ROM; and strength. Shortening ratio is also a predictive factor of worse ADL, with lower values of shortening ratio corresponding to higher values of ADL. To the best of our knowledge, no studies evaluated the RD and RS after F8-B application, hindering the comparison with other studies. The current literature focuses only on ID and IS [48,51–53]. Jones et al. reported that ID is better than IS as a predictor of worse outcomes [54]. Several studies found no association between IS and functional outcomes in agreement with our data outcomes [51,52,55]. Conversely, other studies reported an association between IS and worse outcomes [12,18,39,53,56]. Importantly, two systematic reviews analyzed in detail the impact of IS on the clinical outcomes, concluding that, actually, the published studies do not support an association between the two [49,57]. It should also be pointed out that different methods of measuring clavicle shortening are applied, different immobilization methods are used, as well as different follow-up times, making a comparison between studies difficult.

The present study has several points of weakness and strength. Its main limitations are the retrospective design and the relatively small sample size of a single center. This limitation was due to the choice to enroll only patients who had completed the entire clinical and radiological follow-up and to the strict inclusion criteria. Another limit is the lack of a control group (for example one treated by a simple arm sling), since the study was designed as non-comparative. Furthermore, it could be argued that shoulder position during radiography also has a substantial effect on the length of the fractured clavicle, altering its measurements. However, in our study, the patient was facing toward the radiography film in a standardized way before and after F8-B application to improve the fracture position and to reduce the risks of radiographic bias.

Regarding strengths, our study cohort was a consecutive series of patients treated in our center for an MCF according to our specific, standardized, institutional protocol and followed until fracture healing. Furthermore, contrary to most publications on this subject, displacement and shortening of the fracture were expressed in percentage with respect to the length of the ipsilateral clavicle, after using standardized radiological method to evaluate both displacement and shortening as recommended. This relative measure can be applied to each subject regardless of his or her body characteristics, unlike the expression in length.

To the best of our knowledge, this is the first study that assesses functional outcomes and standardized radiographic aspects (before and after the application of the F8-B) at the time of evaluation in the emergency room, and when evaluating the shortening ratio at last follow-up as well.

Further large-scale, prospective, randomized controlled trials are necessary to better identify those patients in stratified high-risk groups who would be more likely to suffer nonunion and would benefit from early surgery.

5. Conclusions

In conclusion, good to very good mid-term clinical results were obtained managing displaced MCFs of adult patients with conservative treatment according to our institutional protocol. Only a few cases of suboptimal functional scores were recorded, which were attributable to residual clavicular shortening, when severe. In addition, while residual displacement was found to have an impact on fracture healing, residual shortening was a predictor of functional clinical outcomes.

We believe that the findings of this study could be useful for orthopedic surgeons and the treatment should be accurately discussed with patients, explaining the risks and benefits of each therapeutic approach. Finally, the treatment option should be carefully personalized, considering each patient's psycho-physical features, activity level and expectations.

Supplementary Materials: The following are available online at https://www.mdpi.com/article/10.3390/jpm12050759/s1, Table S1: Correlations between clinical outcomes and radiological features; Table S2: Radiological predictors of clinical outcomes (MANCOVA); Figure S1: ROC curve for residual displacement and its impact on CS subscales: pain, ADL, ROM and strength.

Author Contributions: Conceptualization, C.B. and A.P.; methodology, A.P. and E.B.; validation, C.B. and A.B.; formal analysis, N.L.B. and A.P.; investigation, D.S., A.P. and E.B.; resources, C.B., A.B. and P.R.; data curation, A.P. and E.B.; writing-original draft preparation, A.P., E.B. and D.S.; writing-review and editing, A.P., E.B., D.S. and C.B.; visualization, A.P.; supervision, C.B., A.B. and P.R.; project administration, C.B. and P.R. All authors have read and agreed to the published version of the manuscript.

Funding: This research received no external funding.

Institutional Review Board Statement: The study was conducted in accordance with the Declaration of Helsinki, and approved by the Institutional Ethics Committee of University-Hospital of Padova (protocol code CESC code 189N/AO/21, 16 December 2021).

Informed Consent Statement: Informed consent was obtained from all subjects involved in the study.

Data Availability Statement: Data are available contacting the corresponding authors on reasonable request.

Acknowledgments: The authors also thank Jacopo Tagliapietra and Filippo Zonta for their assistance in data collection.

Conflicts of Interest: The authors declare no conflict of interest.

References

1. Postacchini, F.; Gumina, S.; De Santis, P.; Albo, F. Epidemiology of clavicle fractures. *J. Shoulder Elb. Surg.* **2002**, *11*, 452–456. [CrossRef] [PubMed]
2. Robinson, C.M. Fractures of the clavicle in the adult. Epidemiology and classification. *J. Bone Joint Surg. Br.* **1998**, *80*, 476–484. [CrossRef] [PubMed]
3. Coppa, V.; Dei Giudici, L.; Cecconi, S.; Marinelli, M.; Gigante, A. Midshaft clavicle fractures treatment: Threaded Kirschner wire versus conservative approach. *Strateg. Trauma Limb Reconstr.* **2017**, *12*, 141–150.
4. Faldini, C.; Nanni, M.; Leonetti, D.; Acri, F.; Galante, C.; Luciani, D.; Giannini, S. Nonoperative treatment of closed displaced midshaft clavicle fractures. *J. Orthop. Traumatol.* **2010**, *11*, 229–236. [CrossRef] [PubMed]
5. DeFroda, S.F.; Lemme, N.; Kleiner, J.; Gil, J.; Owens, B.D. Incidence and mechanism of injury of clavicle fractures in the NEISS database: Athletic and non athletic injuries. *J. Clin. Orthop. Trauma* **2019**, *10*, 954–958. [CrossRef]
6. Guerra, E.; Previtali, D.; Tamborini, S.; Filardo, G.; Zaffagnini, S.; Candrian, C. Midshaft Clavicle Fractures: Surgery Provides Better Results as Compared With Nonoperative Treatment: A Meta-analysis. *Am. J. Sports Med.* **2019**, *47*, 3541–3551. [CrossRef]
7. Van der Meijden, O.A.; Gaskill, T.R.; Millett, P.J. Treatment of clavicle fractures: Current concepts review. *J. Shoulder Elb. Surg.* **2012**, *21*, 423–429. [CrossRef]
8. Lenza, M.; Belloti, J.C.; Andriolo, R.B.; Gomes Dos Santos, J.B.; Faloppa, F. Conservative interventions for treating middle third clavicle fractures in adolescents and adults. *Cochrane Database Syst. Rev.* **2009**, *12*, CD007121. [CrossRef]
9. Xu, J.; Xu, L.; Xu, W.; Gu, Y. Operative versus nonoperative treatment in the management of midshaft clavicular fractures: A meta-analysis of randomized controlled trials. *J. Shoulder Elb. Surg.* **2014**, *23*, 173–181. [CrossRef]
10. McKnight, B.; Heckmann, N.; Hill, J.R.; Pannell, W.C.; Mostofi, A.; Omid, R.; Hatch, G.F., 3rd. Surgical management of midshaft clavicle nonunions is associated with a higher rate of short-term complications compared with acute fractures. *J. Shoulder Elb. Surg.* **2016**, *25*, 1412–1417. [CrossRef]
11. Martetschläger, F.; Gaskill, T.R.; Millett, P.J. Management of clavicle nonunion and malunion. *J. Shoulder Elb. Surg.* **2013**, *22*, 862–868. [CrossRef] [PubMed]
12. McKee, R.C.; Whelan, D.B.; Schemitsch, E.H.; McKee, M.D. Operative versus nonoperative care of displaced midshaft clavicular fractures: A meta-analysis of randomized clinical trials. *J. Bone Joint Surg. Am.* **2012**, *94*, 675–684. [CrossRef] [PubMed]
13. Robinson, C.M.; Goudie, E.B.; Murray, I.R.; Jenkins, P.J.; Ahktar, M.A.; Read, E.O.; Foster, C.J.; Clark, K.; Brooksbank, A.J.; Arthur, A.; et al. Open reduction and plate fixation versus nonoperative treatment for displaced midshaft clavicular fractures: A multicenter, randomized, controlled trial. *J. Bone Joint Surg. Am.* **2013**, *95*, 1576–1584. [CrossRef] [PubMed]
14. Woltz, S.; Stegeman, S.A.; Krijnen, P.; van Dijkman, B.A.; van Thiel, T.P.; Schep, N.W.; de Rijcke, P.A.; Frölke, J.P.; Schipper, I.B. Plate Fixation Compared with Nonoperative Treatment for Displaced Midshaft Clavicular Fractures: A Multicenter Randomized Controlled Trial. *J. Bone Joint Surg. Am.* **2017**, *99*, 106–112. [CrossRef]
15. Wolf, S.; Chitnis, A.S.; Manoranjith, A.; Vanderkarr, M.; Plaza, J.Q.; Gador, L.V.; Holy, C.E.; Sparks, C.; Lambert, S.M. Surgical treatment, complications, reoperations, and healthcare costs among patients with clavicle fracture in England. *BMC Musculoskelet. Disord.* **2022**, *23*, 135. [CrossRef]
16. Biz, C.; Tagliapietra, J.; Angelini, A.; Belluzzi, E.; Pozzuoli, A.; Berizzi, A.; Ruggieri, P. The challenging management of a delayed union midshaft clavicle fracture complicated by an acute pseudoaneurysm of the subclavian artery in a superelderly diabetic patient. *Aging Clin. Exp. Res.* **2019**, *31*, 567–569. [CrossRef]
17. Ahmed, A.F.; Salameh, M.; AlKhatib, N.; Elmhiregh, A.; Ahmed, G.O. Open Reduction and Internal Fixation Versus Nonsurgical Treatment in Displaced Midshaft Clavicle Fractures: A Meta-Analysis. *J. Orthop. Trauma* **2018**, *32*, e276–e283. [CrossRef]
18. Subramanyam, K.N.; Mundargi, A.V.; Gopakumar, K.U.; Bharath, T.; Prabhu, M.V.; Khanchandani, P. Displaced midshaft clavicle fractures in adults—Is non-operative management enough? *Injury* **2021**, *52*, 493–500. [CrossRef]
19. Amer, K.; Smith, B.; Thomson, J.E.; Congiusta, D.; Reilly, M.C.; Sirkin, M.S.; Adams, M.R. Operative Versus Nonoperative Outcomes of Middle-Third Clavicle Fractures: A Systematic Review and Meta-Analysis. *J. Orthop. Trauma* **2020**, *34*, e6–e13. [CrossRef]
20. Axelrod, D.E.; Ekhtiari, S.; Bozzo, A.; Bhandari, M.; Johal, H. What Is the Best Evidence for Management of Displaced Midshaft Clavicle Fractures? A Systematic Review and Network Meta-analysis of 22 Randomized Controlled Trials. *Clin. Orthop. Relat. Res.* **2020**, *478*, 392–402. [CrossRef]
21. Schneider, P.; Bransford, R.; Harvey, E.; Agel, J. Operative treatment of displaced midshaft clavicle fractures: Has randomised control trial evidence changed practice patterns? *BMJ Open* **2019**, *9*, e031118. [CrossRef] [PubMed]
22. Kluijfhout, W.P.; Tutuhatunewa, E.D.; van Olden, G.D.J. Plate fixation of clavicle fractures: Comparison between early and delayed surgery. *J. Shoulder Elb. Surg.* **2020**, *29*, 266–272. [CrossRef] [PubMed]
23. Potter, J.M.; Jones, C.; Wild, L.M.; Schemitsch, E.H.; McKee, M.D. Does delay matter? The restoration of objectively measured shoulder strength and patient-oriented outcome after immediate fixation versus delayed reconstruction of displaced midshaft fractures of the clavicle. *J. Shoulder Elb. Surg.* **2007**, *16*, 514–518. [CrossRef] [PubMed]
24. Sawalha, S.; Guisasola, I. Complications associated with plate fixation of acute midshaft clavicle fractures versus non-unions. *Eur. J. Orthop. Surg. Traumatol.* **2018**, *28*, 1059–1064. [CrossRef] [PubMed]

25. Virtanen, K.J.; Remes, V.; Pajarinen, J.; Savolainen, V.; Björkenheim, J.M.; Paavola, M. Sling compared with plate osteosynthesis for treatment of displaced midshaft clavicular fractures: A randomized clinical trial. *J. Bone Joint Surg. Am.* **2012**, *94*, 1546–1553. [CrossRef]
26. Tamaoki, M.J.S.; Matsunaga, F.T.; Costa, A.; Netto, N.A.; Matsumoto, M.H.; Belloti, J.C. Treatment of Displaced Midshaft Clavicle Fractures: Figure-of-Eight Harness Versus Anterior Plate Osteosynthesis: A Randomized Controlled Trial. *J. Bone Joint Surg. Am.* **2017**, *99*, 1159–1165. [CrossRef]
27. Van der Ven Denise, J.C.; Timmers, T.K.; Flikweert, P.E.; Van Ijseldijk, A.L.; van Olden, G.D. Plate fixation versus conservative treatment of displaced midshaft clavicle fractures: Functional outcome and patients' satisfaction during a mean follow-up of 5 years. *Injury* **2015**, *46*, 2223–2229. [CrossRef]
28. Jørgensen, A.; Troelsen, A.; Ban, I. Predictors associated with nonunion and symptomatic malunion following non-operative treatment of displaced midshaft clavicle fractures—A systematic review of the literature. *Int. Orthop.* **2014**, *38*, 2543–2549. [CrossRef]
29. Tagliapietra, J.; Belluzzi, E.; Biz, C.; Angelini, A.; Fantoni, I.; Scioni, M.; Bolzan, M.; Berizzi, A.; Ruggieri, P. Midshaft Clavicle Fractures Treated Nonoperatively Using Figure-of-Eight Bandage: Are Fracture Type, Shortening, and Displacement Radiographic Predictors of Failure? *Diagnostics* **2020**, *10*, 788. [CrossRef]
30. Padulo, J.; Oliva, F.; Frizziero, A.; Maffulli, N. Basic principles and recommendations in clinical and field science research: 2018 update. *Muscles Ligaments Tendons J.* **2018**, *8*, 305–307. [CrossRef]
31. Delaune, L.A.; Wehrli, L.; Maeder, Y.; Vauclair, F.; Moerenhout, K. Acute brachial plexus deficit due to clavicle fractures. *JSES Int.* **2021**, *5*, 46–50. [CrossRef] [PubMed]
32. Della Santa, D.; Narakas, A.; Bonnard, C. Late lesions of the brachial plexus after fracture of the clavicle. *Ann. Chir. Main Memb. Super.* **1991**, *10*, 531–540. [CrossRef] [PubMed]
33. Feriani, N.; Ben Ghezala, H.; Snouda, S. Pneumothorax Caused by an Isolated Midshaft Clavicle Fracture. *Case Rep. Emerg. Med.* **2016**, *2016*, 2409894. [CrossRef] [PubMed]
34. Amer, K.M.; Congiusta, D.V.; Suri, P.; Choudhry, A.; Otero, K.; Adams, M. Clavicle fractures: Associated trauma and morbidity. *J. Clin. Orthop. Trauma* **2021**, *13*, 53–56. [CrossRef] [PubMed]
35. Hani, R.; Ennaciri, B.; Jeddi, I.; El Bardouni, A.; Mahfoud, M.; Berrada, M.S. Pneumothorax complicating isolated clavicle fracture. *Pan Afr. Med. J.* **2015**, *21*, 202. [CrossRef]
36. Mouzopoulos, G.; Stamatakos, M.; Arabatzi, H.; Tzurbakis, M. Complications of clavicle fracture and acromioclavicular joint rupture. What the general surgeon should know. *Chirurgia* **2008**, *103*, 509–512.
37. Fletcher, C.; Fletcher, K.L. A delayed and recurrent pneumothorax complicating a fractured clavicle—A novel presentation. *Trauma Case Rep.* **2020**, *26*, 100294. [CrossRef]
38. Gandham, S.; Nagar, A. Delayed pneumothorax following an isolated clavicle injury. *BMJ Case Rep.* **2013**, *2013*, bcr1120115168. [CrossRef]
39. Society, C.O.T. Nonoperative treatment compared with plate fixation of displaced midshaft clavicular fractures. A multicenter, randomized clinical trial. *J. Bone Joint Surg. Am.* **2007**, *89*, 1–10.
40. Ateş, C.; Kaymaz, Ö.; Kale, H.E.; Tekindal, M.A. Comparison of Test Statistics of Nonnormal and Unbalanced Samples for Multivariate Analysis of Variance in terms of Type-I Error Rates. *Comput. Math. Methods Med.* **2019**, *2019*, 2173638. [CrossRef]
41. Wu, C.L.; Chang, H.C.; Lu, K.H. Risk factors for nonunion in 337 displaced midshaft clavicular fractures treated with Knowles pin fixation. *Arch. Orthop. Trauma Surg.* **2013**, *133*, 15–22. [CrossRef] [PubMed]
42. Liu, W.; Xiao, J.; Ji, F.; Xie, Y.; Hao, Y. Intrinsic and extrinsic risk factors for nonunion after nonoperative treatment of midshaft clavicle fractures. *Orthop. Traumatol. Surg. Res.* **2015**, *101*, 197–200. [CrossRef] [PubMed]
43. Clement, N.D.; Goudie, E.B.; Brooksbank, A.J.; Chesser, T.J.; Robinson, C.M. Smoking status and the Disabilities of the Arm Shoulder and Hand score are early predictors of symptomatic nonunion of displaced midshaft fractures of the clavicle. *Bone Joint J.* **2016**, *98-B*, 125–130. [CrossRef] [PubMed]
44. Ziegler, P.; Kühle, L.; Stöckle, U.; Wintermeyer, E.; Stollhof, L.E.; Ihle, C.; Bahrs, C. Evaluation of the Constant score: Which is the method to assess the objective strength? *BMC Musculoskelet. Disord.* **2019**, *20*, 403. [CrossRef]
45. Robertson, G.A.; Wood, A.M. Return to sport following clavicle fractures: A systematic review. *Br. Med. Bull.* **2016**, *119*, 111–128. [CrossRef]
46. Woltz, S.; Krijnen, P.; Schipper, I.B. Mid-Term Patient Satisfaction and Residual Symptoms After Plate Fixation or Nonoperative Treatment for Displaced Midshaft Clavicular Fractures. *J. Orthop. Trauma* **2018**, *32*, e435–e439. [CrossRef]
47. Tutuhatunewa, E.D.; Stevens, M.; Diercks, R.L. Clinical outcomes and predictors of patient satisfaction in displaced midshaft clavicle fractures in adults: Results from a retrospective multicentre study. *Injury* **2017**, *48*, 2788–2792. [CrossRef]
48. Postacchini, R.; Gumina, S.; Farsetti, P.; Postacchini, F. Long-term results of conservative management of midshaft clavicle fracture. *Int. Orthop.* **2010**, *34*, 731–736. [CrossRef]
49. Malik, S.S.; Tahir, M.; Jordan, R.W.; Malik, S.S.; Saithna, A. Is shortening of displaced midshaft clavicle fractures associated with inferior clinical outcomes following nonoperative management? A systematic review. *J. Shoulder Elb. Surg.* **2019**, *28*, 1626–1638. [CrossRef]
50. Moverley, R.; Little, N.; Gulihar, A.; Singh, B. Current concepts in the management of clavicle fractures. *J. Clin. Orthop. Trauma* **2020**, *11*, S25–S30. [CrossRef]

51. Figueiredo, G.S.; Tamaoki, M.J.; Dragone, B.; Utino, A.Y.; Netto, N.A.; Matsumoto, M.H.; Matsunaga, F.T. Correlation of the degree of clavicle shortening after non-surgical treatment of midshaft fractures with upper limb function. *BMC Musculoskelet. Disord.* **2015**, *16*, 151. [CrossRef] [PubMed]
52. Rasmussen, J.V.; Jensen, S.L.; Petersen, J.B.; Falstie-Jensen, T.; Lausten, G.; Olsen, B.S. A retrospective study of the association between shortening of the clavicle after fracture and the clinical outcome in 136 patients. *Injury* **2011**, *42*, 414–417. [CrossRef] [PubMed]
53. Fuglesang, H.F.; Flugsrud, G.B.; Randsborg, P.H.; Stavem, K.; Utvåg, S.E. Radiological and functional outcomes 2.7 years following conservatively treated completely displaced midshaft clavicle fractures. *Arch. Orthop. Trauma Surg.* **2016**, *136*, 17–25. [CrossRef]
54. Jones, G.L.; Bishop, J.Y.; Lewis, B.; Pedroza, A.D. Intraobserver and interobserver agreement in the classification and treatment of midshaft clavicle fractures. *Am. J. Sports Med.* **2014**, *42*, 1176–1181. [CrossRef] [PubMed]
55. Goudie, E.B.; Clement, N.D.; Murray, I.R.; Lawrence, C.R.; Wilson, M.; Brooksbank, A.J.; Robinson, C.M. The Influence of Shortening on Clinical Outcome in Healed Displaced Midshaft Clavicular Fractures After Nonoperative Treatment. *J. Bone Joint Surg. Am.* **2017**, *99*, 1166–1172. [CrossRef] [PubMed]
56. Bajuri, M.Y.; Maidin, S.; Rauf, A.; Baharuddin, M.; Harjeet, S. Functional outcomes of conservatively treated clavicle fractures. *Clinics* **2011**, *66*, 635–639. [CrossRef]
57. Woltz, S.; Sengab, A.; Krijnen, P.; Schipper, I.B. Does clavicular shortening after nonoperative treatment of midshaft fractures affect shoulder function? A systematic review. *Arch. Orthop. Trauma Surg.* **2017**, *137*, 1047–1053. [CrossRef]

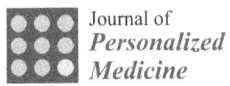

Review

App-Based Rehabilitation in Back Pain, a Systematic Review

Claire Stark [1], John Cunningham [1,2], Peter Turner [1,2], Michael A. Johnson [2] and Henrik C. Bäcker [1,2,*]

1 Department of Orthopaedic Surgery, Royal Melbourne Hospital, 300 Grattan Street, Parkville, VIC 3050, Australia
2 Epworth Richmond Hospital, 89 Bridge Road, Richmond, VIC 3021, Australia
* Correspondence: henrik.baecker@charite.de

Abstract: Smartphones and their associated applications are used frequently by patients and clinicians alike. Despite the technology being widely accessible, their use to aid in rehabilitation is yet to be adopted. The SARS CoV-2 pandemic has presented an opportunity to expedite their integration given the difficulty patients currently have in accessing healthcare. The aim of this study was to perform a systematic literature review on the use of smartphone rehabilitation applications compared to standard physiotherapy for back pain. We conducted a search of Medline/Pubmed and google databases using the search terms [APP] AND [[Orthopaedic] OR [Neurosurgery]], following the PRISMA guidelines. All prospective studies investigating rehabilitation applications for back pain or following spine surgery were included. A total of nine studies met the inclusion criteria which investigated 7636 patients, of which 92.4% were allocated to the interventional group ($n = 7055/7636$) with a follow up of 4 weeks to 6 months. All except one study reported on patients experiencing back pain on average for 19.6 ± 11.6 months. The VAS-pain score was presented in all studies without significance between the interventional and control group ($p = 0.399$ before and $p = 0.277$ after intervention). Only one research group found significantly higher improvement in PROMs for the application group, whereas the remaining showed similar results compared to the control group. Using application-based rehabilitation programs provides an easily accessible alternative or substitute to traditional physiotherapy for patients with back pain. Given that smartphones are so prevalent in activities in our daily lives, this will enhance and improve rehabilitation if patients are self-dedicated and compliant.

Keywords: applications; back; spine; pain; rehabilitation

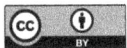

1. Introduction

Rehabilitation is a common feature in patients in the post-operative phase after spinal surgery as well as patients with chronic back pain [1]. Traditionally, these rehabilitation services have been delivered through face-to-face consultation with patients. Since the advent of SARS-CoV2, there has been a prompt turn to the digitalisation of the provision of healthcare [2]. The pandemic has highlighted the advantages of remote rehabilitation programs delivered through a smartphone device.

Smartphone ownership worldwide surpassed 6 billion in July 2022 [3]. In 2021 in the United States, over a third of the population's media time was spent on mobile phones, and 72.3% of that was on smartphones [4]. The significant utilisation of smartphones and their apps provides an opportunity to integrate their use into clinical practice and help reduce the barriers patients face in accessing health care.

Apps are increasingly used in healthcare, streamlining communication, recording patient outcome data and in some cases measuring outcome data. A survey of 146 patients in a neurosurgical waiting room found that 81% of patients (whom had not had previous surgery) expressed interest in using a postoperative communication and monitoring app [5]. A 2015 study found that there were 72 individual spine surgery-themed apps, of which 45 were free to download; however, only 56% had named medical professionals involved in their development or content [6].

There is evidence supporting telerehabilitation in general orthopaedics [7]; however, there is a void when specifically referring to app-based rehabilitation in back pain and following spine surgery. This systematic review aims to summarize the existing literature and data reporting the outcomes of app-based rehabilitation programs in back pain and following spine surgery.

2. Materials and Methods

A systematic review was performed on the 30 July 2022. The Pubmed/MEDLINE, Cochrane and Google Scholar databases were searched following the Preferred Reporting Items for Systematic Reviews and Meta-Analyses (PRISMA) guidelines [8]. The search terms included [APP] AND [[Orthopaedic] OR [Neurosurgery]], which were thought to be the broadest terms. All studies were included that presented their results in English, German or French, analysing the outcome of smartphone app-based rehabilitation in back pain patients and those following spine surgery. Non-accessible full articles, letters to the editors and comments were excluded, as well as those which failed to present functional outcome following rehabilitation.

Applying the PICO scheme, our objective included the comparison of control versus interventional group (O, C) in patients with low back pain (P, I). Hereby, we assumed that the app-based rehabilitation is at least as efficient as general physiotherapy (C, O).

The quality of publications as well as the risk of bias was assessed (Table 1). Data on population demorahics such as including age, gender, duration of back pain, body mass index (BMI), indication, follow up, patient reported outcome measures (PROM) and apps used were recorded. As functional outcomes, the visual analogue scale of pain (VAS), SF-36, Likert score, PHQ-9, Korff and current symptom score (CSS) were used. In addition, the significances presented in the individual studies were noted, comparing the control with the intervention group.

Table 1. Quality assessment results using the risk-of-bias assessment tool.

First Author	Year of Publication	Randomization	Allocation Concealment	Incomplete Outcome Data	Adequate Follow Up	Selective Reporting
Amorim AB	2019	+	-	-	-	-
Bailey JF	2020	-	-	+	-	-
Chhabra HS	2018	+	-	+	-	+
Hasenöhrl T	2020	-	+	+	-	+
Huber S	2017	-	-	-	-	-
Irvine AB	2015	+	-	-	-	+
Shebib R	2019	+	+	+	-	-
Toelle TR	2019	+	+	-	-	-
Yang J	2019	+	-	+	-	+

SPSS (SPSS, Inc., IBM Company, Chicago, IL, USA) and Microsoft Excel (Microsoft Corporation, Redmond, WA, USA) were applied for statistical analyses. Data are presented as absolute numbers and percentages and significances are set to p-values < 0.05.

Using our search terms, a total of 1122 articles were found and screened for inclusion criteria. Overall, 91 articles were duplicates and a total of 105 articles were screened. One article needed to be exluded as it analyzed postoperative recovery without specifying the surgery [9]. In total, 9 articles were included in the final analysis (Figure 1).

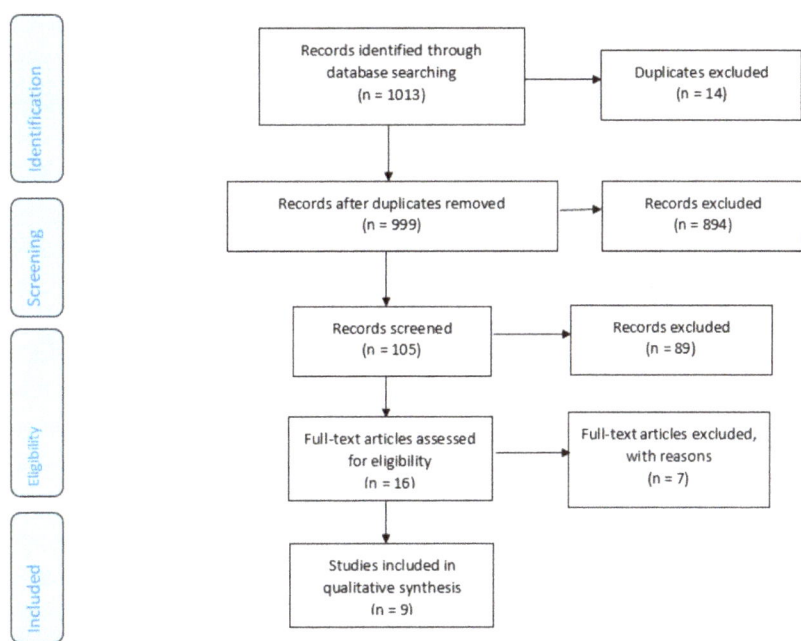

Figure 1. Included articles according to the PRISMA Guidelines.

3. Results

Within the 9 prospective studies, 7636 patients were investigated, of which 466 were assigned to the control group. Irvine AB et al. also included an alternative group ($n = 199$), leaving 7055 patients in the interventional group. The mean age was 44.2 ± 7.4 years, and the majority of patients were females (75.3%, $n = 5638/7487$). Where BMI was included, the mean was 26.3 ± 2.2 kg/m^2, and the pain duration reported was 19.6 ± 11.6 months. All findings are presented in Table 2.

Some authors reported on chronic lower back pain, others reported on back and neck pain [10], and lastly on non-specific back pain [11]. All studies lacked detailed definitions, raising questions regarding the aetiology of the aforementioned pain.

Smartphone applications included the Kaya App [12,13], Snapcare [14], Fitbit app [15] or FitBack [16]. In the remaining studies, the app used was not specified. Follow up varied from 4 weeks [11] to 6 months [15]. Not only did the follow up presentation differ between the groups, but also the presentation of the results.

The only consistent patient reported outcome measure was the visual analogue scale of pain at rest, which was 4.9 ± 1.2 for the interventional group and 5.2 ± 1.2 for the control group. This improved in the long term to 3.1 ± 1.0 and 3.6 ± 0.5, respectively. However, no significant differences were found between the two groups ($p = 0.399$ before and $p = 0.277$ after intervention).

Seven authors described significant findings ($p < 0.05$). This varied between the pain, vitality [17], physical function and Oswestry score or overall [12,14,16,18]. Irvine et al. further described significant differences between the control and treatment group after 16 weeks. Bailey et al., Huber S et al. and Amorin AB et al. did not report any significant differences. All findings are illustrated in Tables 3 and 4.

Table 2. Demographics of all included study.

First Author	Year of Publication	Intervention	Indication	Number of Patients (n)	Age (Years)	Gender (Female)	Bodyweight (kg)	BMI (kg/m²)	Pain Duration (Months)
Amorim AB	2019	Fitbit app	Chronic low back pain	31	59.5 ± 11.9	15		28.9 ± 6.0	
		Control		24	57.1 ± 14.9	19		27.2 ± 5.1	
Bailey JF	2020	Unspecified app	Neck and Backpain	6468	42.6 ± 10.9	4981		29.8 ± 7.1	
Chhabra HS	2018	Snapcare app	Chronic low back pain	45	41.4 ± 14.2		63.4 ± 12.5	23.2 ± 4.2	22.8 ± 22.0
		Control		48	41.0 ± 14.2		66.2 ± 11.5	23.5 ± 3.8	28.0 ± 25.5
Hasenöhrl T	2020	Unspecified app	Non specific back pain	27			81.7 ± 22.5	28.1 ± 7.1	
Huber S	2017	Kaya app	Low back pain	105	33.9 ± 10.9	105			More than 12 weeks (73.3%)
Irvine AB	2015	Fitback	Low back pain	199		116			
		Alternative care		199		117			
		Control		199		125			
Shebib R	2019	Unspecified app	Back pain	133	43.0 ± 11.0	37%		26.0 ± 5.0	
		Control		64	43.0 ± 12.0	48%		26.0 ± 4.0	
Toelle TR	2019	Kaya App	Chronic low back pain	42	41.0 ± 10.6	35		24.4 ± 3.3	7.2 ± 3.4
		Control		44	43.0 ± 11.0	31		25.4 ± 4.6	6.7 ± 3.1
Yang J	2019	unspecified app	Chronic low back pain	5	35.0 ± 19.3	1	64.8 ± 10.3		35.8 ± 54.4
		Control		3	50.3 ± 9.3	3	62.0 ± 15.9		17.0 ± 17.1
Sum				7636		5548			
Average					44.2 ± 7.4		67.7 ± 7.2	26.3 ± 2.2	19.6 ± 11.6

Table 3. Indication, Oswestry score and VAS of pain; overall means, standard deviations and p-values. R-VAS—visual analogue scale of pain at rest, A-VAS—visual analogue scale of pain during activity, LT—long term, ST—short term.

First Author	Year of Publication	Intervention	Follow Up	ODI Score Before	ODI Score ST	ODI Score LT	R-VAS	ST	LT	A-VAS	ST	LT	Significances
Amorim AB	2019	Fitbit app	6 months				5.3		3.8				$p = 0.815$
		control					5.1		4.0				
Bailey JF	2020	Intervention	12 weeks				4.6		1.4				$p < 0.001$
Chhabra HS	2018	Snapcare	12 weeks				7.3		3.3				$p < 0.05$
		Control					6.6		3.2				
Hasenöhrl T	2020	Unspecified app	4 weeks	17.1	14.4		3.2	3.2					$p < 0.001$
Huber S	2017	Kaya App	12 weeks				4.8	3.2	2.6				$p < 0.001$, between control and treatment
Irvine AB	2015	Fitback	16 weeks				3.0	3.3	3.4				
		Alternative care					3.0	3.3	3.5				
		Control					2.9	3.1	3.3				
Shebib R	2019	Unspecified app	12 weeks	21.7		19.7	4.6		4.4	3.9		3.7	$p < 0.05$
		Control		21.0		18.9	4.5		4.3	4.4		4.1	
Toelle TR	2019	Kaya App	12 weeks				5.1	4.3	2.7				$p = 0.021$
		Control					5.4	4.1	3.4				
Yang J	2019	Unspecified app	4 weeks				5.9	3.4					$p < 0.05$ for vitality
		Control					6.0	6.0					
Sum		Intervention					4.9 ± 1.2	3.5 ± 0.5	3.1 ± 1.0	3.9		3.7	
		Control					5.2 ± 1.2	4.4 ± 1.5	3.6 ± 0.5	4.4		4.1	

Table 4. PROMs following rehabilitation programs for back pain and following spine surgery. Score indicates the PROM used; overall means, standard deviations and *p*-values.

First Author	Year of Publication	Score	Pain			Symptoms/ Emotions/ Other			Function in ADL			Sport/ Recreation			Quality of Life/Vitality			Overall	
				ST	LT		ST	LT		ST	LT		ST	LT		ST	LT		ST
Amorim AB	2019	Likert										202.20		187.70	1984.90		2065.70		
Bailey JF	2020	PHQ-9/Korff	15.95		7.75	4.39						200.50		169.20	1936.70		1941.20		
Chhabra HS	2018	Current Symptom score/SF-36	7.02	3.27		2.11	1.22		4.82	3.02		3.35	1.27		11.56	1.04		52.1	20.2
Hasenöhrl T	2020	SF-36	38.78	53.59		71.26	80.25		65.15	68.41		2.58			2.09				
Huber S	2017	VAS										72.78	77.78		54.44	61.67		41.4	29.2
Irvine AB	2015	Multidimensional Pain Inventory Interference Scale, Dartmouth CO-OP, WLQ	2.96	3.32	3.38	4.02	4.59	4.90	3.63	3.27	3.03	3.14	3.38		3.51				
			3.01	3.30	3.47	4.07	4.48	4.65	3.93	3.45	3.31	3.10	3.34		3.37				
			2.92	3.08	3.28	4.08	4.03	4.12	4.03	3.85	3.74	3.09	3.11		3.14				
Shebib R	2019	VAS	45.53	41.65		44.38	46.53								48.69	50.58			
Toelle TR	2019	SF-36	47.32	40.78		44.56	45.56								47.64	48.64			
Yang J	2019	SF-36	44.00	40.00		58.40	60.07		49.00	50.00		74.00	59.00		50.00	47.00			
			63.33	56.67		66.67	44.56		58.33	65.00		46.67	51.67		63.33	65.00			
Sum		Intervention	42.77 ± 3.54	45.08 ± 7.42		58.01 ± 13.44	62.28 ± 16.97		57.08 ± 11.42	59.21 ± 13.02		73.39 ± 0.86	68.39 ± 13.28		51.04 ± 3.01	53.08 ± 7.65			
		Control	55.33 ± 11.32	48.73 ± 11.25		55.62 ± 15.63	45.06 ± 0.71		58.33	65.00		46.67	51.67		55.49 ± 11.09	56.82 ± 11.57			

4. Discussion

This systematic review shows no significant differences between application-based rehabilitation and standard physiotherapy (control group) in patients who suffer from back pain for a mean of 19.6 ± 11.6 months. In most studies, the pain improved significantly despite the technique of rehabilitation. Due to the heterogeneity of data, a true meta analysis could not be executed.

Applications in healthcare currently include diabetes [19], weight loss [20], mental health [21], speech disorders [22] and cardiovascular diseases [23], which need to be assessed according to the content quality and benchmark the interventions against best practice guidelines.

Adherence to a postoperative rehabilitation program is one of the major barriers to successful app-based rehabilitation [24]. The compliance is typically low and up to 30% fail to attend classes [25,26]. Consistency in program engagement is crucial to achieving a satisfying outcome. In self-motivated patients with high compliance, app-based rehabilitation shows an effective approach for pain improvement. Rather than presenting different exercises, a sensor could be used to give live feedback to the patients, such as measuring the muscle strength applied.

Within the investigated studies, a variety of different apps were used. The Kaya App adopts comprehensive evidence-based multidisciplinary pain treatment following the international disease management guidelines according to the authors [12,13]. Further significantly lower pain intensity scores were found compared to the control group. The app could also be used during the waiting time until patients are admitted to the pain clinic, as it seems to be an effective low-cost treatment without delay [12]. In contrast, the Snapcare app was designed to monitor the patient's daily activity level and symptomatic profile. Thereby, individual home exercises are presented and individual activity goals set. These are selected based on the baseline health data, PROM scores and pain levels which are assessed after each activity session [14]. Likewise, Fitbit monitors the individual goals and physical activates and report on physical activity-related goals. In addition, a health coach gives regular feedback via telephone and able to discuss the participants goals and progress. Further individual healthy tips are provided to the users [15]. According to Irvine et al., FitBack is an online app which provides self-monitoring of cognitive and behavioural strategies to improve self-care and back pain-prevention behaviours Exercises are selected based on safety with minimal equipment which can be performed without supervision [16].

Machado et al. performed a search and found a total of 61 available apps in 2016. The majority offered a combination of biomechanical exercises, yoga or strengthening/stretching. Those which scored the highest number of points recommended a combination of biomechanical exercises including strengthening, stretching, core stability or McKenzie exercises [27]. One weakness outlined was the questionable evidence-based intervention, as the majority had not been tested in a randomized controlled trial. Additionally, the authors mentioned that the app quality did not correlate with the in-app or online user ratings. Therefore, they concluded that the user ratings are invalid indicators of app quality. This may relate to a missing pre-exercise questionnaire assessing preconditions such as comorbidities or previous surgeries. Further, the users may have different experience levels, which should be considered.

There are further considerations to implementing app-based rehabilitation programs in community healthcare. The cost of app download was not mentioned, with some applications requiring a single payment for download, whereas others require a subscription-type model. Additionally, whilst smartphones are prevalent in the general community, the usability and app interface would need to consider the target audience. Finally, whilst an app-based rehabilitation is an exciting development in digital healthcare, the safety of those engaging in an unsupervised activity needs to be forefront of mind. An app would need to consider the risk of certain exercises (i.e., falls) if undertaken alone.

The largest cohort investigating the impact of app-based rehabilitation on back pain included 6468 patients. The authors reported a high completion and engagement rate, providing benefits for the groups. The average improvement in VAS pain was 68.5% within the first 12 weeks, where 78.6% completed the program regularly. For back pain, the standardized mean difference was 1.37, which was the same for both genders. Unfortunately, the study failed to include a control group, and since it was a longitudinal observational study, no detailed findings were presented [10].

There are several limitations to this study. In the search terms, we did not include [physical therapy], as we believed that this would return articles relating to unspecific back pain or nutritional apps. The quality of the individual studies was low (range of bias scores 1–3/5), and therefore a meta-analysis was not completed due to the heterogeneity of the data. However, these studies represent the most important examples in this field. The consistent factor within the studies was the visual analogue scale of pain. Additionally, the time to follow up ranged from only 4 weeks to 6 months. Furthermore, different patient reported outcome measures were used, including SF-36, Likert, the Oswestry Disability Index, current symptoms, PHQ-9, and the Korff score. Finally, it has to be mentioned that chronic back pain may resolve itself over time regardless of the rehabilitation activities performed. However, we would expect a significant difference between the two groups, as rehabilitation activities may hasten the rehabilitation.

5. Conclusions

Application-based rehabilitation for back pain and following spine surgery is as good as standard physiotherapy. Although no significant differences can be found between the two cohorts, application-based rehabilitation's integration into healthcare seems promising, especially in motivated patients who regularly engage in independent rehabilitation. Furthermore, in patients who are unable to visit physiotherapists, such as during pandemics or due to living in rural locations, this is an excellent approach which may further lower healthcare costs.

Author Contributions: Conceptualization, C.S. and H.C.B.; methodology, C.S., H.C.B. and J.C.; software, C.S. and H.C.B.; validation, C.S., J.C. and H.C.B.; formal analysis, C.S. and H.C.B.; investigation, C.S., P.T. and H.C.B.; resources, P.T. and M.A.J.; data curation, C.S. and H.C.B.; writing—original draft preparation, C.S., P.T., M.A.J., J.C. and H.C.B.; writing—review and editing, C.S., P.T., M.A.J., J.C. and H.C.B.; visualization, H.C.B. and J.C.; supervision, C.S. and H.C.B.; project administration, H.C.B. All authors have read and agreed to the published version of the manuscript.

Funding: This research received no external funding.

Institutional Review Board Statement: The study was conducted in accordance with the Declaration of Helsinki. No ethical approval was required for this study.

Informed Consent Statement: N/A because of the systematic review.

Data Availability Statement: Not applicable.

Conflicts of Interest: The authors declare no conflict of interest.

References

1. Madera, M.; Brady, J.; Deily, S.; McGinty, T.; Moroz, L.; Singh, D.; Tipton, G.; Truumees, E. The role of physical therapy and rehabilitation after lumbar fusion surgery for degenerative disease: A systematic review. *J. Neurosurg. Spine* **2017**, *26*, 694–704. [CrossRef] [PubMed]
2. Amankwah-Amoah, J.K.Z.; Wood, G.; Knight, G. COVID-19 and digitalization: The great acceleration. *J. Bus. Res.* **2021**, *136*, 602–611. [CrossRef] [PubMed]
3. O'Dea, S. Smartphone Subscriptions Worldwide 2016–2027. Statista. 2022. Available online: https://www.statista.com/statistics/330695/number-of-smartphone-users-worldwide/ (accessed on 8 June 2022).
4. Dolan, S. How Mobile Users Spend Their Time on Their Smartphones in 2022. eMarketer. 2022. Available online: https://www.insiderintelligence.com/insights/mobile-users-smartphone-usage/#:~{}:text=Mobile%20usage%20statistics,digital%20media%20time%20per%20day (accessed on 8 June 2022).

5. Nathan, J.K.; Rodoni, B.M.; Joseph, J.R.; Smith, B.W.; Park, P. Smartphone Use and Interest in a Spine Surgery Recovery Mobile Application Among Patients in a US Academic Neurosurgery Practice. *Oper. Neurosurg.* **2020**, *18*, 98–102. [CrossRef] [PubMed]
6. Robertson, G.A.J.; Wong, S.J.; Brady, R.R.; Subramanian, A.S. Smartphone apps for spinal surgery: Is technology good or evil? *Eur. Spine J.* **2016**, *25*, 1355–1362. [CrossRef]
7. Petersen, W.; Karpinski, K.; Backhaus, L.; Bierke, S.; Haner, M. A systematic review about telemedicine in orthopedics. *Arch. Orthop. Trauma Surg.* **2021**, *141*, 1731–1739. [CrossRef] [PubMed]
8. Moher, D.; Liberati, A.; Tetzlaff, J.; Altman, D.G.; The PRISMA Group. Preferred reporting items for systematic reviews and meta-analyses: The PRISMA statement. *PLoS Med.* **2009**, *6*, e1000097. [CrossRef]
9. Hou, J.; Yang, R.; Yang, Y.; Tang, Y.; Deng, H.; Chen, Z.; Wu, Y.; Shen, H. The Effectiveness and Safety of Utilizing Mobile Phone–Based Programs for Rehabilitation After Lumbar Spinal Surgery: Multicenter, Prospective Randomized Controlled Trial. *JMIR mHealth uHealth* **2019**, *7*, e10201. [CrossRef]
10. Bailey, J.F.; Agarwal, V.; Zheng, P.; Smuck, M.; Fredericson, M.; Kennedy, D.J.; Krauss, J. Digital Care for Chronic Musculoskeletal Pain: 10,000 Participant Longitudinal Cohort Study. *J. Med. Internet Res.* **2020**, *22*, e18250. [CrossRef]
11. Hasenöhrl, T.; Windschnurer, T.; Dorotka, R.; Ambrozy, C.; Crevenna, R. Prescription of individual therapeutic exercises via smartphone app for patients suffering from non-specific back pain: A qualitative feasibility and quantitative pilot study. *Wien. Klin. Wochenschr.* **2020**, *132*, 115–123. [CrossRef]
12. Toelle, T.R.; Utpadel-Fischler, D.A.; Haas, K.-K.; Priebe, J.A. App-based multidisciplinary back pain treatment versus combined physiotherapy plus online education: A randomized controlled trial. *NPJ Digit. Med.* **2019**, *3*, 1–9. [CrossRef]
13. Huber, S.; A Priebe, J.; Baumann, K.-M.; Plidschun, A.; Schiessl, C.; Tölle, T.R. Treatment of Low Back Pain with a Digital Multidisciplinary Pain Treatment App: Short-Term Results. *JMIR Rehabil. Assist. Technol.* **2017**, *4*, e11. [CrossRef]
14. Chhabra, H.S.; Sharma, S.; Verma, S. Smartphone app in self-management of chronic low back pain: A randomized controlled trial. *Eur. Spine J.* **2018**, *27*, 2862–2874. [CrossRef]
15. Amorim, A.B.; Pappas, E.; Simic, M.; Ferreira, M.L.; Tiedemann, A.; Jennings, M.; Ferreira, P. Integrating Mobile health and Physical Activity to reduce the burden of Chronic low back pain Trial (IMPACT): A pilot trial protocol. *BMC Musculoskelet. Disord.* **2016**, *17*, 36. [CrossRef]
16. Irvine, A.B.; Russell, H.; Manocchia, M.; Mino, D.E.; Glassen, T.C.; Morgan, R.; Gau, J.M.; Birney, A.J.; Ary, D.V.; Buhrman, M.; et al. Mobile-Web App to Self-Manage Low Back Pain: Randomized Controlled Trial. *J. Med. Internet Res.* **2015**, *17*, e1. [CrossRef]
17. Yang, J.; Wei, Q.; Ge, Y.; Meng, L.; Zhao, M. Smartphone-Based Remote Self-Management of Chronic Low Back Pain: A Preliminary Study. *J. Healthc. Eng.* **2019**, *2019*, 1–7. [CrossRef]
18. Shebib, R.; Bailey, J.F.; Smittenaar, P.; Perez, D.A.; Mecklenburg, G.; Hunter, S. Randomized controlled trial of a 12-week digital care program in improving low back pain. *Npj Digit. Med.* **2019**, *2*, 1–8. [CrossRef]
19. Arnhold, M.; Quade, M.; Kirch, W. Mobile Applications for Diabetics: A Systematic Review and Expert-Based Usability Evaluation Considering the Special Requirements of Diabetes Patients Age 50 Years or Older. *J. Med. Internet Res.* **2014**, *16*, e104. [CrossRef]
20. Mateo, G.F.; Granado-Font, E.; Ferré-Grau, C.; Montaña-Carreras, X. Mobile Phone Apps to Promote Weight Loss and Increase Physical Activity: A Systematic Review and Meta-Analysis. *J. Med. Internet Res.* **2015**, *17*, e253. [CrossRef]
21. Lee, H.; Sullivan, S.J.; Schneiders, A.; Ahmed, O.H.; Balasundaram, A.P.; Williams, D.; Meeuwisse, W.H.; McCrory, P. Smartphone and tablet apps for concussion road warriors (team clinicians): A systematic review for practical users. *Br. J. Sports Med.* **2014**, *49*, 499–505. [CrossRef]
22. Furlong, L.M.; Morris, M.E.; Erickson, S.; Serry, T.A.; Robles-Bykbaev, V.; Amlani, A.M. Quality of Mobile Phone and Tablet Mobile Apps for Speech Sound Disorders: Protocol for an Evidence-Based Appraisal. *JMIR Res. Protoc.* **2016**, *5*, e233. [CrossRef]
23. Santo, K.; Richtering, S.S.; Chalmers, J.; Thiagalingam, A.; Chow, C.K.; Redfern, J. Mobile Phone Apps to Improve Medication Adherence: A Systematic Stepwise Process to Identify High-Quality Apps. *JMIR mHealth uHealth* **2016**, *4*, e132. [CrossRef]
24. Argent, R.; Daly, A.; Caulfield, B. Patient Involvement With Home-Based Exercise Programs: Can Connected Health Interventions Influence Adherence? *JMIR mHealth uHealth* **2018**, *6*, e47. [CrossRef]
25. McGregor, A.H.; Henley, A.; Morris, T.P.; Doré, C.J. An Evaluation of a Postoperative Rehabilitation Program After Spinal Surgery and Its Impact on Outcome. *Spine* **2012**, *37*, E417–E422. [CrossRef]
26. Johnson, R.E.; Jones, G.T.; Wiles, N.J.; Chaddock, C.; Potter, R.G.; Roberts, C.; Symmons, D.; Watson, P.J.; Torgerson, D.; Macfarlane, G. Active exercise, education, and cognitive behavioral therapy for persistent disabling low back pain: A randomized controlled tria. *Spine* **2007**, *32*, 1578–1585. [CrossRef]
27. Machado, G.C.; Pinheiro, M.B.; Lee, H.; Ahmed, O.H.; Hendrick, P.; Williams, C.; Kamper, S.J. Smartphone apps for the self-management of low back pain: A systematic review. *Best Pract. Res. Clin. Rheumatol.* **2016**, *30*, 1098–1109. [CrossRef]

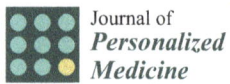

Review

A Review of Functional Outcomes after the App-Based Rehabilitation of Patients with TKA and THA

Henrik Constantin Bäcker [1,2,*], Chia H. Wu [3], Dominik Pförringer [4], Wolf Petersen [5], Ulrich Stöckle [1] and Karl F. Braun [4,5]

[1] Charité—Universitätsmedizin Berlin, Corporate Member of Freie Universität Berlin and Center for Musculoskeletal Surgery, Humboldt-Universität zu Berlin, Charitéplatz 1, 10117 Berlin, Germany
[2] Royal Melbourne Hospital, Department of Orthopedic Surgery, 300 Grattan Street, Parkville, VIC 3050, Australia
[3] Department of Orthopedics & Sports Medicine, Baylor College of Medicine Medical Centre, Houston, TX 77030, USA
[4] Klinik und Poliklinik für Unfallchirurgie, Klinikum Rechts der Isar der TU München, Ismaninger Street 22, 81675 München, Germany
[5] Department of Orthopedics, Martin Luther Hospital, Berlin-Grunewald, Caspar-Theyß-Straße 27-31, 14193 Berlin, Germany
* Correspondence: henrik.baecker@charite.de

Abstract: Following the outbreak of SARS-CoV-2, several elective surgeries were cancelled, and rehabilitation units were closed. This has led to difficulties for patients seeking access to rehabilitation in order to achieve the best possible outcome. New applications with or without sensors were developed to address this need, but the outcome has not been examined in detail yet. The aim of this study was to perform a systematic literature review on smart phone applications for patients suffering from hip and knee osteoarthritis after arthroplasty. The MEDLINE/PubMed and Google databases were queried using the search term "[APP] AND [ORTHOPEDIC]" according to PRISMA guidelines. All prospective studies investigating rehabilitation applications reporting the functional outcome in hip and knee osteoarthritis after arthroplasty were included. The initial search yielded 420 entries, but only 9 publications met the inclusion criteria, accounting for 1067 patients. In total, 518 patients were in the intervention group, and 549 patients were in the control group. The average follow-up was 9.5 ± 8.1 months (range: 3 to 23.4 months). Overall, significantly lower A-VAS values were observed for the interventional group in the short term ($p = 0.002$). There were no other significant differences observed between the two groups. Smart phone applications provide an alternative to in-person sessions that may improve access for patients after total joint arthroplasty. Our study found there are significant improvements in the short term by using this approach. In combination with a blue-tooth-enabled sensor for isometric exercises, patients can even receive real-time feedback after total knee arthroplasty.

Keywords: applications; knee; hip; osteoarthritis; rehabilitation

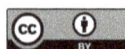

1. Introduction

Since the inception of the SARS-CoV-2 pandemic, digitalization has progressed rapidly around the world [1,2]. Social distancing has contributed to a reduction in elective surgeries in orthopedic surgery and has decreased access to postop rehabilitation for arthroplasty patients [3]. This may have led to worse outcomes and delayed returns to activity. Additionally, restrictions in the range of motion are likely to be present, resulting in major limitations. Although digital surgical approaches involving virtual and augmented reality, as well as robot navigation systems, have become increasingly popular, there is a lack of digital rehabilitation programs. With the number of smartphone users worldwide estimated to reach 3.8 billion by 2021 [4], there is an opportunity to deliver physical therapy easily at relatively low costs. Bahadori et al. recently published a systematic review, showing that there are 15 applications available on smartphone app stores focusing on rehabilitation following total hip and knee arthroplasty. However, these varied significantly in their quality and outlined a missing partnership with patients. Therefore, the authors questioned the clinical importance [5]. In a further study, the evidence supporting the use of smartphone apps and wearable devices was assessed. Here, wearable devices were capable of monitoring physical activity and improving patient engagement following total knee arthroplasty [6]. Both of these reviews, however, failed to report the functional outcome in detail.

In addition, telemedicine, virtual digital scribes, chat bots and surgical scheduling applications for consultations have all reportedly led to new improvements in patient care [7]. For digital rehabilitation, telehealth visits with a live video feed in conjunction with a physical therapist are still the most common. To date, physical therapy delivered entirely via smart phone applications lacks evidence. In 2019, Campbell et al. showed that patients receiving automated text messages after total joint arthroplasty led to an increased amount of time spent on home exercises. This also leads to improvements in the patient's mood and a decreased use of narcotics, while minimizing calls to the surgeon's office [8].

Besides home training reminders delivered via text messages, an app-based approach offers a variety of different individual training programs; this can allow a blue-tooth-enabled sensor to be connected to provide real-time feedback. This has the potential to improve compliance, as it is more convenient logistically, especially for immobilized patients. Furthermore, cost and wait times can be reduced. This study aims to summarize the published data on using this approach to provide postoperative rehabilitation for hip and knee arthroplasty patients.

2. Materials and Methods

A systematic literature review was conducted on 25 April 2022, searching the MEDLINE, Cochrane and Google scholar databases. The Preferred Reporting Items for Systematic Reviews and Meta-Analyses (PRIMSA) guidelines were followed (Figure 1) [9].

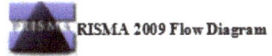

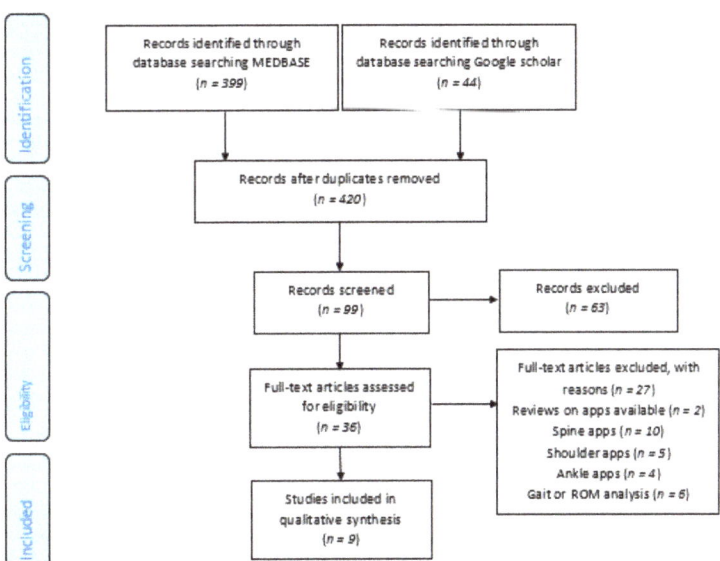

Figure 1. Included articles according to the PRISMA Guidelines.

The broadest inclusive terms were applied to include all relevant studies. We used the search term "[APP] AND [Orthopedic]" and included all full articles in English, German and French. The analysis was performed by a fellowship-trained orthopedic surgeon and a sports medicine physician. We only included prospective studies that investigated application-based rehabilitation programs in patients suffering from knee and hip osteoarthritis, as well as those who had undergone total hip and knee arthroplasty. We excluded retrospective studies, letters to the editor and comments or studies that are not full articles. Studies that lack a functional outcome were also excluded.

For each study that met the inclusion criteria, the number of patients, gender, age, comorbidities, length of hospitalization, follow-up, body mass index (BMI), indication (knee vs hip osteoarthritis), patient-reported outcome measures (PROM) and apps used with or without a sensor were analyzed. Regarding functional outcome, changes in endurance tests within six minutes, changes in walking speed, changes in functional mobility, the time up to go (TUG) test, the five times sit to stand test (FSST), the hip disability and osteoarthritis outcome score (HOOS), the knee injury and osteoarthritis outcome score (KOOS) and the SF-36 survey were recorded. Other outcome measures include the Knee society score (KSS), visual analogue scale at rest as well as activity (R-VAS/A-VAS), range of motion (ROM), Western Ontario, McMaster Universities Osteoarthritis Index (WOMAC), Euro Quality of Life (EQ-5D-3L), short questionnaire to assess health-enhancing physical activity (SQUASH) and patient activation measure (PAM-13).

For statistical analysis, SPSS (SPSS, Inc., IBM Company, Chicago, IL, USA) and Microsoft Excel (Microsoft Corporation, Redmond, DC, USA) were used. All data are presented in absolute numbers and percentages; significances are set to p-values < 0.05. Because of the heterogeneity of the data, we were not able to perform a meta-analysis.

3. Results

Our search terms revealed a total of 420 entries. A total of 99 publications investigated the application-based rehabilitation, of which 36 publications investigated either hip or knee osteoarthritis in the context of total knee or hip arthroplasty. A total of 27 articles were excluded, leaving 9 publications for the final analysis.

Within the 9 studies, 1067 patients were analyzed, including 518 patients in the intervention group and 549 patients in the control group. The mean age was 63.3 ± 3.5 years, and 41.8% of patients were male ($n = 384/919$). The mean BMI was 29.5 ± 2.3 kg/m^2, and patients suffered from 3 ± 2.3 comorbidities, on average. The mean length of hospital stay was reported to be 9.1 ± 4.2 days, and the average follow-up was 9.5 ± 8.1 months (range 3 to 23.4 months). For rehabilitation programs, four authors reported that a sensor or motion tracker was used, whereas an app-based exercise instruction was delivered via a smartphone or a tablet in the remaining five studies. All of the included studies are illustrated in Table 1.

For total knee arthroplasty, four studies were included [10–13]. Three of the four studies reported the KOOS score [10–12]. Two of the studies reported the long-term outcome, whereas only one reported the functional outcome after a one-week follow-up [11]. Van Dijk-Huisman reported the standing and walking times and the functional recovery [13]. Only one study presented the TUG, HOOS and SF-36 scores [14]. In the remaining four studies, patients suffered from knee [15] and hip osteoarthritis [16–18]. Those studies reported the changes in the functional mobility, timed up to go test, disability and functional independence measure [16], self-management behavior [17] and visual analogue scale at rest (R-VAS) [18].

Table 1. Included studies and demographics of patients included.

Author	Year	No. Patients	Age (Year)	Gender (Male) (No.)	BMI (kg/m^2)	Follow-Up (Months)	Digital Program	Indication	Hospital Stay (Days)	Days of Intervention	Comorbidities (No.)
Arfaei Chitkar SS	2021	31	57.84		27.97		Application instruction	Knee osteoarthritis		56	7
Control group		29	58.52		26.62					56	5
Bäcker HC	2021	20	62.95	8	32.33	23.73	Application with sensor	TKA	6.6		1
Control group		15	66.27	6	33.79	23.35			6.9		1
Correia FD	2019	38	67.3	32	31.0	6	Application with motion tracker	TKA	6.0	56	Detailed listing
Control group		31	70.0	22	30.8	6			6.0	56	Detailed listing
Hardt S	2018	22	63.3	10	31.6	7	Application with sensor	TKA	6.6	6.6	1
Control group		25	67.6	10	32.4	7			6.9	6.9	1
Li I	2020	44	65				Application instruction	Arthritis	14.7	14.7	4
Control group		44	66						14.2	14.2	4
Pelle T	2020	214	62.1	67	27.8		Application instruction	Osteoarthritis			
Control group		213	62.1	54	27.3						
Skrepnik N	2017	107	61.6	48	29.4	3	Application with sensor	Osteoarthritis			
Control group		104	63.6	57	29.3	3					
Control group		61	66.0	40	27.73						
Van Dijk-Huisman HC	2020	27	65.1	15	27.47		Application with sensor	TKA		31	
Control group		61	66.0	40	27.73					31	
Wijnen A	2020	15	59.3	5	26.7	6	Application instruction	THA		84	
Control group		15	59.3	5	28					84	
Control group		12	59.3	5	31.1					84	
Intervention group		518	62.7 + 2.9	443 (41.8%)	29.3 + 2.1	9.2 + 8.3			9.1 + 4.9		3.3 + 2.9
Control group		549	63.9 + 3.9	467 (41.8%)	29.7 + 2.5	9.8 + 9.2			9.0 + 4.5		2.8 + 2.1
p-value			0.243	0.449	0.368	0.454			0.493		0.393

Although higher KOOS scores were found in the short term as well as the long term, no overall significances were found. Following THA, Wijnen described significantly higher HOOS scores for function in sport and recreational activities and hip-related quality of life. This is also observed for the SF-36 physical role limitations at 12 weeks and 6 months post-surgery [12]. The overall A-VAS score was significantly lower in the app-based group in the short term ($p = 0.002$). Notably, both of these studies were published by the same group of authors [10,11]. All PROMs and results are presented in Table 2. Furthermore, no significant differences between the individual indications and the application with or without sensors were identified.

Table 2. PROMs following rehabilitation programs for knee/hip osteoarthritis, as well as following joint replacement. Score indicates the PROM used; overall means, standard deviations and p-values were calculated for HOOS/KOOS and self-management behavior scores, as these are comparable. Empty cells—not reported in the individual studies. N/A—not applicable. Significances presented in bold.

	No. Patients	Six-Minute Endurance ST	Walking Speed (10 min) ST	Change in Disability ST	Score	Pain ST	Pain LT	Symptoms ST	Symptoms LT	Function in ADL ST	Function in ADL LT	Sport/Recreation ST	Sport/Recreation LT	Quality of Life ST	Quality of Life LT	R-VAS ST	R-VAS LT	A-VAS ST	A-VAS LT
Arfaei Chakar SS	31				WOMAC	18.5		5.6		48.3									
Control group	29				WOMAC	17.2		5.6		49.6									
Bäcker HC	20		11.77	19.66	KOOS	42.4	81.7	50.6		61.7	64.5	54.6	77.2	16.0	9.5	48.6	18.4	26.7	68.4
Control group	15		12.39	27.08	KOOS	37.8	80.7	48.6		63.1	61.6	51.0	77.1	9.3	8.1	47.3	14.2	30.8	67.9
Correia FD	38				KOOS	33.0	95.5	34.0	100.0	51.5	96.0	93.0	97.0	0	30.0	42.5	13.0	81.0	94.0
Control group	31				KOOS	47.0	86.0	50.0	86.0	82.0	86.0	87.0	87.0	5.0	20.0	20.0	25.0	56.0	63.0
Hardt S	22	0.9		0.6	KOOS	45.0		62.0		60.0		54.0		14.0	10.0		17.0	30.0	
Control group	25	0.8		0.5	KOOS	36.0		58.0		59.0		42.0		12.0	5.0		18.0	26.0	
Li J	44	delta = 115.6	delta = 0.4	17.3	Self-management behavior														
Control group	44	delta = 103.3	delta = 0.4	18.0	Self-management behavior														
Pelle T	214					57.5	59.4	57.7		57.3	57.3	58.5	62.1	32.6	31.9	33.4	38.0		
Control group	213					58.2	57.5	57.0		56.2	55.2	59.4	58.6	32.5	33.2	33.2	38.3		
Skorpnik N	107	402.8			18.2														
Control group	104	395.6			6.3														
Van Dijk-Huisman HC	27				Standing walking time/functional recovery					70.9		−0.3							
Wijnen A	15				HOOS	48.9	88.8	50.0		75.3	91.0	103.0	96.8	1.0	70.0	82.5	19.2	50.8	88.8
Control group	15				HOOS	35.5	85.1	29.3		68	76.3	52.7	80	23.3	26.7	59.6	22.9	45.8	71.3

	R-VAS ST	R-VAS LT	A-VAS ST	A-VAS LT
Bäcker HC	3.6	2.7	7.6	4.0	2.7
Control group	4.3	3.6	6.7	5.1	2.8
Hardt S	4.0	2.0	7.0	4.0
Control group	4.0	4.0	7.0	5.0
Pelle T	4.6	2.7		
Control group	5.1	3.6		
Skorpnik N	delta = −55.3			
Control group	delta = −33.8			

Table 2. Cont.

	No. Patients	Six-Minute Endurance		Walking Speed (10 min)		Change in Disability		Score	Pain		Symptoms		Function in ADL		Sport/Recreation		Quality of Life		R-VAS		A-VAS	
		ST	LT	ST	LT	ST	LT		ST	LT	ST	LT	ST	LT	ST	LT	ST	LT	ST	LT	ST	LT
Control group	12	402.8	N/A	6.34	10.13	17.3	118.2	HOOS	36.3	77.5	41.7	85.6	62.1	77.5	37.1	58.1	79.1	20.8	29.7	64.9	24.5	43.2	69.3	4.07	2.35	0.9	7.3	4	2.7
Intervention group Std.	518	N/A	N/A	7.69	13.48	N/A	N/A		45.36	7.16	50.86	84.95	61.16	77.2	47.6	67.9	83.275	17.18	30.28	51.75	21.12	40.36	67.88	0.50	0.49	N/A	0.42	0	N/A
Control group Std.	549	395.6	N/A	6.60	13.79	18.0	N/A		8.97	19.36	10.68	18.96	8.80	19.16	9.13	16.71	16.90	12.06	24.61	21.43	9.73	12.04	3.54	4.47	3.8	0.9	6.85	5.05	2.8
		N/A	N/A	8.20	18.79	N/A	N/A		41.80	63.30	47.43	78.98	65.07	71.32	41.88	99.53	76.36	15.98	20.45	45	23.82								
p-value		N/A	N/A	0.977	0.844	N/A	N/A		9.12	14.00	10.70	12.20	9.20	12.58	8.97	15.09	10.61	9.77	11.65	18.57	8.23								
									0.532	1.574	0.609	0.583	0.493	0.595	0.324	0.405	0.475	0.899	0.405	0.628	0.630	0.607	0.069	0.413	0.069	N/A	0.312	0.002	N/A

4. Discussion

This review shows that patients can benefit from digital apps for the rehabilitation of osteoarthritis in the context of total joint arthroplasty, especially for the short term (A-VAS). In the long term, no statistical significances were observed, although the values for the app-based groups were slightly higher overall. Despite the different applications investigated, with or without the use of sensors, no correlations were found.

For rehabilitation, total knee arthroplasty is easier to investigate, as weakness in the flexors or extensors can be measured. The hip is much more complex, as the rotators, flexors, extensors and abductors all need to be strengthened and can be difficult to assess individually. However, overall function can still be assessed, with the six-minute endurance test and walking speed as examples.

The development of applications and digital platforms is typically associated with high fixed costs and lower variable costs. Once an application is developed and operational in a market, the marginal cost of treating an additional patient is quite low and thus more scalable. However, insurance coverage for app-based therapy is still very limited [19].

Although significant improvements were observed in the short term, no significant differences were found in the long term. Digital apps can be another tool when there is no access to in-person rehabilitation following total knee arthroplasty. The addition of blue tooth sensors in total knee arthroplasty can provide real-time feedback to patients in order to motivate them. Other indications have already been investigated in sports medicine and following cruciate ligament replacements [20,21]. In particular, isometric exercises can be effectively performed this way. Eccentric and concentric movements are much more difficult to simulate, as they typically require in-person supervision. Sensors can also detect dynamic valgus malalignment, which is one of the main risk factors for anterior cruciate ligament injury and re-injury [22].

A disadvantage of this approach is that the history of injuries, previous surgeries or comorbidities may not be built into the workout program. Likewise, other factors such as surgical techniques (e.g., cemented vs. non-cemented THA, CR TKA vs. PS TKA) are typically not taken into account. Furthermore, the poor fitting and calibration of sensors can potentially provide misleading feedback for patients. This may call for a combined approach where initial sessions are instructed in person and then transition to an app-based approach with careful remote monitoring by a qualified provider to adapt the training as required. While regular text messages or push notifications can help to improve compliance, some degree of motivation is still required to use the app effectively [8]. Finally, it must be mentioned that elderly patients may have difficulty navigating smart devices and may not be willing to use applications if they prefer in-person sessions.

The app-based delivery of care is promising, and the data summarized in our study support its use. With the help of artificial intelligence and a thorough initial assessment regarding individual comorbidities, individual limitations and preoperative conditions, a personalized training/rehabilitation algorithm can be developed. This will improve the effectivity of training and, subsequently, compliance and satisfaction. In conjunction with robotic navigation, augmented reality, virtual reality and artificial intelligence can potentially optimize outcomes and improve efficiency. The different questionnaires and patient-reported outcome measures seen in the various studies included in our systemic review are difficult to compare. In addition, an individual's motivation and compliance to app instructions are not measured in these studies. As such, it is difficult to delineate exactly how often the individual apps were used by the patients.

There are several limitations to this study. As this one is a review, the analysis depends on the individual studies. Additionally, as we only searched the PubMed/Medbase and Google Scholar databases, some articles that were published on EMBASE or the Web of Science, along with grey literature, may have been missed. Further, no quality assessment was performed. For outcomes, the rehabilitation monitored was not further specified, and, subsequently, no recommendations were made. Finally, as the data were heterogenic, we were not able to perform a meta-analysis.

5. Conclusions

Digital applications provide a good adjunctive tool for rehabilitation following total joint arthroplasty, with significant improvements in the short term. After total knee arthroplasty, isometric exercises in particular can be performed with a sensor to allow for real-time feedback. Eccentric and concentric exercises are more difficult to perform via this approach. We do not believe that this new technology replaces physiotherapists, but it will more likely serve as another tool in our armamentarium. With proper instruction, applications can help and motivate patients, ideally with regular follow-ups to see if adjustments are required.

Author Contributions: Conceptualization, K.F.B. and H.C.B.; methodology, K.F.B., H.C.B. and U.S.; software, H.C.B.; validation, K.F.B., C.H.W. and H.C.B.; formal analysis, H.C.B.; investigation, K.F.B., C.H.W. and H.C.B.; resources, U.S. and W.P.; data curation, D.P. and H.C.B.; writing—original draft preparation, K.F.B., C.H.W., U.S., W.P., D.P. and H.C.B.; writing—review and editing, K.F.B., C.H.W., U.S., W.P., D.P. and H.C.B.; visualization, H.C.B. and K.F.B.; supervision, U.S. and H.C.B.; project administration, H.C.B. All authors have read and agreed to the published version of the manuscript.

Funding: This research received no external funding.

Institutional Review Board Statement: The study was conducted in accordance with the Declaration of Helsinki. No ethical approval was required for this study.

Informed Consent Statement: Not applicable.

Data Availability Statement: Not applicable.

Acknowledgments: We acknowledge the support from the German Research Foundation (DFG) and the Open Access Publication Funds of Charité—Universitätsmedizin Berlin.

Conflicts of Interest: The authors declare no conflict of interest.

References

1. Amankwah-Amoah, J.; Khan, Z.; Wood, G.; Knight, G. COVID-19 and digitalization: The great acceleration. *J. Bus. Res.* **2021**, *136*, 602–611. [CrossRef] [PubMed]
2. Petersen, W.; Karpinski, K.; Backhaus, L.; Bierke, S.; Haner, M. A systematic review about telemedicine in orthopedics. *Arch. Orthop. Trauma. Surg.* **2021**, *141*, 1731–1739. [CrossRef] [PubMed]
3. The Lancet, R. Too long to wait: The impact of COVID-19 on elective surgery. *Lancet Rheumatol* **2021**, *3*, e83. [CrossRef]
4. Statista.com. Number of Smartphone Users Worldwide from 2016 to 2021. Available online: https://www.statista.com/statistics/330695/number-of-smartphone-users-worldwide/ (accessed on 1 April 2022).
5. Bahadori, S.; Wainwright, T.W.; Ahmed, O.H. Smartphone apps for total hip replacement and total knee replacement surgery patients: A systematic review. *Disabil. Rehabil.* **2020**, *42*, 983–988. [CrossRef]
6. Constantinescu, D.; Pavlis, W.; Rizzo, M.; Berge, D.V.; Barnhill, S.; Hernandez, V.H. The role of commercially available smartphone apps and wearable devices in monitoring patients after total knee arthroplasty: A systematic review. *EFORT Open Rev.* **2022**, *7*, 481–490. [CrossRef]
7. Bini, S.A.; Schilling, P.L.; Patel, S.P.; Kalore, N.V.; Ast, M.P.; Maratt, J.D.; Schuett, D.J.; Lawrie, C.M.; Chung, C.C.; Steele, G.D. Digital Orthopaedics: A Glimpse Into the Future in the Midst of a Pandemic. *J. Arthroplast.* **2020**, *35*, S68. [CrossRef]
8. Campbell, K.J.; Louie, P.K.; Bohl, D.D.; Edmiston, T.; Mikhail, C.; Li, J.; Khorsand, D.A.; Levine, B.R.; Gerlinger, T.L. A Novel, Automated Text-Messaging System Is Effective in Patients Undergoing Total Joint Arthroplasty. *JBJS* **2019**, *101*, 145–151. [CrossRef]
9. Moher, D.; Liberati, A.; Tetzlaff, J.; Altman, D.G.; Group, P. Preferred reporting items for systematic reviews and meta-analyses: The PRISMA statement. *PLoS Med.* **2009**, *6*, e1000097. [CrossRef]
10. Backer, H.C.; Wu, C.H.; Schulz, M.R.G.; Weber-Spickschen, T.S.; Perka, C.; Hardt, S. App-based rehabilitation program after total knee arthroplasty: A randomized controlled trial. *Arch. Orthop. Trauma. Surg.* **2021**, *141*, 1575. [CrossRef]
11. Hardt, S.; Schulz, M.R.G.; Pfitzner, T.; Wassilew, G.; Horstmann, H.; Liodakis, E.; Weber-Spickschen, T.S. Improved early outcome after TKA through an app-based active muscle training programme-a randomized-controlled trial. *Knee Surg. Sports Traumatol. Arthrosc.* **2018**, *26*, 3429. [CrossRef]
12. Correia, F.D.; Nogueira, A.; Magalhaes, I.; Guimaraes, J.; Moreira, M.; Barradas, I.; Molinos, M.; Teixeira, L.; Tulha, J.; Seabra, R.; et al. Medium-Term Outcomes of Digital Versus Conventional Home-Based Rehabilitation after Total Knee Arthroplasty: Prospective, Parallel-Group Feasibility Study. *JMIR Rehabil. Assist. Technol.* **2019**, *6*, e13111. [CrossRef]
13. van Dijk-Huisman, H.C.; Weemaes, A.T.R.; Boymans, T.; Lenssen, A.F.; de Bie, R.A. Smartphone App with an Accelerometer Enhances Patients' Physical Activity Following Elective Orthopedic Surgery: A Pilot Study. *Sensors* **2020**, *20*, 4317. [CrossRef]

14. Wijnen, A.; Hoogland, J.; Munsterman, T.; Gerritsma, C.L.; Dijkstra, B.; Zijlstra, W.P.; Dekker, J.S.; Annegarn, J.; Ibarra, F.; Slager, G.E.; et al. Effectiveness of a Home-Based Rehabilitation Program After Total Hip Arthroplasty Driven by a Tablet App and Remote Coaching: Nonrandomized Controlled Trial Combining a Single-Arm Intervention Cohort With Historical Controls. *JMIR Rehabil. Assist. Technol.* **2020**, *7*, e14139. [CrossRef]
15. Arfaei Chitkar, S.S.; Mohaddes Hakkak, H.R.; Saadati, H.; Hosseini, S.H.; Jafari, Y.; Ganji, R. The effect of mobile-app-based instruction on the physical function of female patients with knee osteoarthritis: A parallel randomized controlled trial. *BMC Women's Health* **2021**, *21*, 333. [CrossRef]
16. Li, I.; Bui, T.; Phan, H.T.; Llado, A.; King, C.; Scrivener, K. App-based supplemental exercise in rehabilitation, adherence, and effect on outcomes: A randomized controlled trial. *Clin. Rehabil.* **2020**, *34*, 1083–1093. [CrossRef]
17. Pelle, T.; Bevers, K.; van der Palen, J.; van den Hoogen, F.H.J.; van den Ende, C.H.M. Effect of the dr. Bart application on healthcare use and clinical outcomes in people with osteoarthritis of the knee and/or hip in the Netherlands; a randomized controlled trial. *Osteoarthr. Cartil.* **2020**, *28*, 418–427. [CrossRef]
18. Skrepnik, N.; Spitzer, A.; Altman, R.; Hoekstra, J.; Stewart, J.; Toselli, R. Assessing the Impact of a Novel Smartphone Application Compared With Standard Follow-Up on Mobility of Patients With Knee Osteoarthritis Following Treatment With Hylan G-F 20: A Randomized Controlled Trial. *JMIR Mhealth Uhealth* **2017**, *5*, e7179. [CrossRef]
19. Gomes, M.; Murray, E.; Raftery, J. Economic Evaluation of Digital Health Interventions: Methodological Issues and Recommendations for Practice. *Pharmacoeconomics* **2022**, *40*, 367. [CrossRef]
20. Wong, S.J.; Robertson, G.A.; Connor, K.L.; Brady, R.R.; Wood, A.M. Smartphone apps for orthopaedic sports medicine-a smart move? *BMC Sports Sci. Med. Rehabil.* **2015**, *7*, 23. [CrossRef]
21. Rathleff, M.S.; Bandholm, T.; McGirr, K.A.; Harring, S.I.; Sorensen, A.S.; Thorborg, K. New exercise-integrated technology can monitor the dosage and quality of exercise performed against an elastic resistance band by adolescents with patellofemoral pain: An observational study. *J. Physiother.* **2016**, *62*, 159–163. [CrossRef]
22. Petersen, W.; Ellermann, A.; Gosele-Koppenburg, A.; Best, R.; Rembitzki, I.V.; Bruggemann, G.P.; Liebau, C. Patellofemoral pain syndrome. *Knee Surg. Sports Traumatol. Arthrosc.* **2014**, *22*, 2264–2274. [CrossRef] [PubMed]

MDPI
St. Alban-Anlage 66
4052 Basel
Switzerland
www.mdpi.com

Journal of Personalized Medicine Editorial Office
E-mail: jpm@mdpi.com
www.mdpi.com/journal/jpm

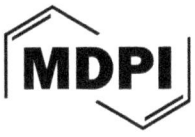

Disclaimer/Publisher's Note: The statements, opinions and data contained in all publications are solely those of the individual author(s) and contributor(s) and not of MDPI and/or the editor(s). MDPI and/or the editor(s) disclaim responsibility for any injury to people or property resulting from any ideas, methods, instructions or products referred to in the content.

www.ingramcontent.com/pod-product-compliance
Lightning Source LLC
LaVergne TN
LVHW070603100526
838202LV00012B/550